Neurologic Manifestations of Rheumatic Diseases

Editors

SARAH E. GOGLIN
JOHN B. IMBODEN

RHEUMATIC DISEASE CLINICS OF NORTH AMERICA

www.rheumatic.theclinics.com

Consulting Editor
MICHAEL H. WEISMAN

November 2017 • Volume 43 • Number 4

ELSEVIER

1600 John F. Kennedy Boulevard • Suite 1800 • Philadelphia, Pennsylvania, 19103-2899
http://www.theclinics.com

RHEUMATIC DISEASE CLINICS OF NORTH AMERICA Volume 43, Number 4
November 2017 ISSN 0889-857X, ISBN 13: 978-0-323-54901-1

Editor: Lauren Boyle
Developmental Editor: Casey Potter

Rheumatic Disease Clinics of North America (ISSN 0889-857X) is published quarterly by Elsevier Inc., 360 Park
Avenue South, New York, NY 10010-1710. Months of issue are February, May, August, and November. Business
and editorial offices: 1600 John F. Kennedy Boulevard, Suite 1800, Philadelphia, PA 19103-2899. Periodicals
postage paid at New York, NY and additional mailing offices. Subscription prices are USD 335.00 per year for
US individuals, USD 659.00 per year for US institutions, USD 100.00 per year for US students and residents,
USD 395.00 per year for Canadian individuals, USD 823.00 per year for Canadian institutions, USD 465.00 per
year for international individuals, USD 823.00 per year for international institutions, and USD 230.00 per year
for Canadian and foreign students/residents. To receive student/resident rate, orders must be accompanied
by name of affiliated institution, date of term, and the *signature* of program/residency coordinator on institution
letterhead. Orders will be billed at individual rate until proof of status received. Foreign air speed delivery is included in all *Clinics* subscription prices. All prices are subject to change without notice. **POSTMASTER:** Send
address changes to *Rheumatic Disease Clinics of North America,* Elsevier Health Sciences Division, Subscription
Customer Service, 3251 Riverport Lane, Maryland Heights, MO 63043. **Customer Service: 1-800-654-2452 (US
and Canada). From outside of the US and Canada: 314-447-8871. Fax: 314-447-8029. For print support,
e-mail: JournalsCustomerService-usa@elsevier.com. For online support, e-mail: JournalsOnline
Support-usa@elsevier.com.**

Reprints. For copies of 100 or more of articles in this publication, please contact the Commercial Reprints
Department, Elsevier Inc., 360 Park Avenue South, New York, New York, 10010-1710; Tel.: +1-212-633-
3874, Fax: +1-212-633-3820, and E-mail: reprints@elsevier.com.

Rheumatic Disease Clinics of North America is covered in *MEDLINE/PubMed (Index Medicus), Current
Contents/Clinical Medicine, Science Citation Index, ISI/BIOMED,* and *EMBASE/Excerpta Medica.*

Contributors

CONSULTING EDITOR

MICHAEL H. WEISMAN, MD
Cedars-Sinai Chair in Rheumatology, Director, Division of Rheumatology, Professor of Medicine, Cedars-Sinai Medical Center, Distinguished Professor, David Geffen School of Medicine at UCLA, Los Angeles, California, USA

EDITORS

SARAH E. GOGLIN, MD
Assistant Professor of Medicine, Division of Rheumatology, UCSF School of Medicine, San Francisco, California, USA

JOHN B. IMBODEN, MD
Alice Betts Endowed Chair for Research in Arthritis, Professor, Division of Rheumatology, Department of Medicine, UCSF School of Medicine, Chief, Zuckerberg San Francisco General Hospital and Trauma Center, San Francisco, California, USA

AUTHORS

MAHMOUD ABDELRAZEK, MD
Rheumatology Unit, Massachusetts General Hospital, Boston, Massachusetts, USA

MICHAEL J. BRADSHAW, MD
Fellow, Partners Multiple Sclerosis Center, Brigham and Women's Hospital, Massachusetts General Hospital, Boston, Massachusetts, USA

TRACEY A. CHO, MD, MA
Associate Professor, Department of Neurology, Massachusetts General Hospital, Boston, Massachusetts, USA

FELICIA C. CHOW, MD, MAS
Assistant Professor, Department of Neurology and Division of Infectious Diseases, University of California, San Francisco, San Francisco, California, USA

SHARON A. CHUNG, MD, MAS
Division of Rheumatology, Russell/Engleman Rheumatology Research Center, University of California, San Francisco, San Francisco, California, USA

KIMBERLY DeQUATTRO, MD
Fellow, Division of Rheumatology, Department of Medicine, University of California, San Francisco, San Francisco, California, USA

SARAH E. GOGLIN, MD
Assistant Professor of Medicine, Division of Rheumatology, UCSF School of Medicine, San Francisco, California, USA

JONATHAN GRAF, MD
Professor of Medicine, University of California, San Francisco, Division of Rheumatology, Zuckerberg San Francisco General Hospital and Trauma Center, San Francisco, California, USA

JOHN B. IMBODEN, MD
Alice Betts Endowed Chair for Research in Arthritis, Professor, Division of Rheumatology, Department of Medicine, UCSF School of Medicine, Chief, Zuckerberg San Francisco General Hospital and Trauma Center, San Francisco, California, USA

KASHIF JAFRI, MD
Division of Rheumatology, Department of Medicine, University of California, San Francisco, San Francisco, California, USA

CRISTINA LANATA, MD
Division of Rheumatology, Department of Medicine, University of California, San Francisco, San Francisco, California, USA

JENNIFER MANDAL, MD
Division of Rheumatology, Russell/Engleman Rheumatology Research Center, University of California, San Francisco, San Francisco, California

MARY MARGARETTEN, MD, MAS
Associate Professor of Medicine, Division of Rheumatology, University of California, San Francisco, San Francisco, California, USA

ERIC L. MATTESON, MD, MPH
Division of Rheumatology, Department of Internal Medicine, Division of Epidemiology, Department of Health Science Research, Mayo Clinic College of Medicine & Science, Rochester, Minnesota, USA

SARAH L. PATTERSON, MD
Division of Rheumatology, Department of Medicine, University of California, San Francisco, San Francisco, California, USA

JOHN H. STONE, MD, MPH
Rheumatology Unit, Massachusetts General Hospital, Boston, Massachusetts, USA

PATOMPONG UNGPRASERT, MD
Division of Rheumatology, Department of Internal Medicine, Mayo Clinic College of Medicine & Science, Rochester, Minnesota, USA; Division of Rheumatology, Department of Medicine, Faculty of Medicine Siriraj Hospital, Mahidol University, Bangkok, Thailand

Contents

measurements, cerebrospinal fluid findings, specific neuroimaging findings, and exclusion of alternative causes. Current treatment encompasses the identification and management of the inciting event, symptomatic treatment, and anticoagulation or immunosuppression.

Neurologic manifestations are common in patients with antiphospholipid antibodies and include stroke, seizures, dementia, cognitive dysfunction, chorea, migraine, psychosis, and demyelinating disease. Many of these disorders mimic their idiopathic counterparts, but treatment of antiphospholipid antibody–associated disease can be different from the treatment of central nervous system disease not associated with these antibodies. For patients with antiphospholipid antibody–associated neurologic disease, anticoagulation or immunosuppressive therapy or both may significantly improve their symptoms. Thus, clinicians should have a high index of suspicion for antiphospholipid syndrome in the appropriate clinical context.

Neurologic manifestations of rheumatoid arthritis (RA) range in severity from mild paresthesias in the hand from carpal tunnel syndrome to sudden death caused by impingement of the medulla by an eroded, vertically subluxed dens. Most neurologic complications are a consequence of articular inflammation and damage that leads to compression of adjacent structures of the central or peripheral nervous systems. Rare but serious extra-articular manifestations include inflammation of the meninges and ischemic neuropathies caused by necrotizing arteritis of the vasa vasorum. Medical therapy with synthetic disease-modifying antirheumatic drugs and biologic agents has diminished the incidence of serious neurologic manifestations in RA.

Central nervous system (CNS) disease is an uncommon but significant complication of granulomatosis with polyangiitis (GPA) and microscopic polyangiitis (MPA) and affects 3 primary areas of the CNS: the pituitary, the pachymeninges, and the CNS vasculature. Pituitary disease is uncommon, but hormonal deficiencies can be long lasting even if there is excellent disease response. Chronic hypertrophic pachymeningitis occurs in patients positive for anti–proteinase 3 with systemic GPA and in antimyeloperoxidase-positive patients with a milder and more limited form of the disease. Cerebral and spinal vasculitis caused by GPA and MPA presents with focal and general neurologic abnormalities.

Neuromyelitis optica, formerly known as Devic disease, is an autoimmune astrocytopathic disease characterized by transverse myelitis and optic neuritis. Most patients have a relapsing course with incomplete recovery between attacks, resulting in progressive disability. The pathogenesis involves production of aquaporin-4 immunoglobulin G (AQP4-IgG) antibodies by plasmablasts in peripheral circulation, disruption of the blood-brain barrier, complement-mediated astrocyte injury, and secondary demyelination. The diagnosis relies on characteristic clinical manifestations in the presence of serum AQP4-IgG positivity or specific neuroimaging findings, and exclusion of alternative causes. Current treatment involves aggressive immunosuppression with pulse-dose steroids during acute attacks and long-term immunosuppression for attack prevention.

Neurosarcoidosis occurs in 3% to 10% of patients with sarcoidosis. Cranial neuropathy and meningeal involvement are the most common manifestations, but any part of the nervous system can be affected. Definite diagnosis requires the presence of noncaseating granuloma in the nervous system, although histopathologic confirmation is often not obtainable. Moderate to high doses of glucocorticoids is the main therapy for neurosarcoidosis. Relapse often occurs after the dose of glucocorticoids is tapered down, often necessitating the use of steroid-sparing immunosuppressive agents.

Patients on immunosuppressive therapy for rheumatic diseases are at increased risk of infection. Although infections of the central nervous system (CNS) are less common compared with other sites, patients on broadly immunosuppressive and biologic immunomodulatory agents may be susceptible to more severe, disseminated forms of infection, including of the CNS. Certain key principles regarding infection risk apply across immunosuppressive therapies, including increased risk with higher doses and longer duration of therapy and with combination therapy. Providers should be aware of the CNS infection risk related to immunosuppressant use to help guide best practices for screening and prophylaxis.

Immunoglobulin G4–related disease (IgG4-RD) can involve nearly any organ system, including the central and peripheral nervous systems. IgG4 antibodies are not known to play a primary causal role in disease. IgG4-RD must be distinguished from a growing number of immune-mediated conditions in which IgG4 autoantibodies contribute directly to pathophysiology. The most common neurologic features of IgG4-RD result from disease in the orbits, pachymeninges, and substance of the pituitary gland and stalk, as well as a perineuropathy that can involve peripheral or cranial nerves. Disease affecting the brain parenchyma is rare but has been reported.

Peripheral nerve involvement is common in polyarteritis nodosa and the
antineutrophil cytoplasmic antibody (ANCA)–associated vasculitides. The
underlying mechanism is arteritis of the vasa nervorum, leading to
ischemic neuropathy. The classic presentation is stepwise involvement
of peripheral nerves with ongoing antecedent constitutional symptoms.
This article reviews the pathologic findings, clinical syndromes, diagnosis,
and treatment of ANCA-associated vasculitides.

RHEUMATIC DISEASE CLINICS
OF NORTH AMERICA

THE CLINICS ARE AVAILABLE ONLINE!
Access your subscription at:
www.theclinics.com

Foreword

Neurologic Manifestations of Rheumatic Diseases

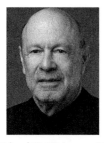

Michael H. Weisman, MD
Consulting Editor

As Sarah Goglin and John Imboden point out, neurologic manifestations of rheumatic diseases often represent sources of confusion and quandary resulting in delay of diagnosis and institution of management. The purpose of this issue is to clarify as much as possible the latest advances in our understanding of these challenges and to place them in a format that is user-friendly for the rheumatologist. Sarah and John have done a truly remarkable job here. All our inflammatory rheumatic diseases have neurologic manifestations, and from a historical perspective, these manifestations may have dominated the clinical picture in years past (such as in rheumatoid arthritis and lupus) but are seen less commonly today. This issue provides a unique challenge for our trainees, who may not have a chance to see, during their fellowship training, some of these patients. That is why the approach by Sarah and John is so important because an issue of this nature with its perspective from these excellent clinicians can embolden a young clinician to face these challenges.

Michael H. Weisman, MD
Division of Rheumatology
Cedars-Sinai Medical Center
David Geffen School of Medicine at UCLA
8700 Beverly Boulevard
Los Angeles, CA 90024, USA

E-mail address:
Michael.Weisman@cshs.org

http://dx.doi.org/10.1016/j.rdc.2017.08.002
0889-857X/17/© 2017 Published by Elsevier Inc.
rheumatic.theclinics.com

Preface

Neurologic Manifestations of Rheumatic Diseases

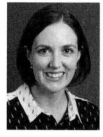 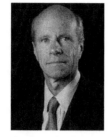

Sarah E. Goglin, MD   John B. Imboden, MD
Editors

Among the most challenging clinical problems faced by rheumatologists are the accurate diagnosis and proper treatment of the neurologic manifestations of systemic rheumatic diseases. It is with this general concept in mind that we chose the topics for review in this issue of *Rheumatic Disease Clinics of North America*.

Several articles focus on entities that have been clearly defined only in the past decade or so. Among these is neuromyelitis optica, once known as Devic disease and poorly understood, but now recognized to be an autoimmune disease associated with autoantibodies to aquaporin 4, a water channel protein. Similarly, the last decade has seen remarkable progress in the characterization of the protean manifestations of IgG4-related disease, now known to have important central nervous system (CNS) involvement. Advances in imaging and astute clinical observation underscore the complexity of primary CNS vasculitis and have led to the recognition and characterization of an important mimicker of vasculitis: reversible cerebral vasoconstriction syndrome.

Rheumatologists have long grappled with neurologic involvement in systemic lupus erythematosus, primary Sjogren syndrome, and sarcoidosis, and these entities are covered here in detail. There has been growing appreciation of the neurologic manifestations of antiphospholipid antibody syndrome, a topic reviewed in this issue, including recognition that some clinical syndromes may be due to direct effects of antiphospholipid antibodies rather than the consequence of thromboembolic events. Because effective control of rheumatoid arthritis appears to have reduced the incidence of complications of the disease, many current practitioners may not have a working knowledge of the neurologic manifestations reviewed here. Finally, the wide spread of

Rheum Dis Clin N Am 43 (2017) xiii–xiv
http://dx.doi.org/10.1016/j.rdc.2017.08.001
0889-857X/17/© 2017 Published by Elsevier Inc.

rheumatic.theclinics.com

effective immunosuppressive therapies has come at the cost of increased infections, including ones that affect the CNS and that also are reviewed here.

Sarah E. Goglin, MD
University of California–San Francisco
Box 0326
San Francisco, CA 94143, USA

John B. Imboden, MD
Division of Rheumatology
Zuckerberg San Francisco General Hospital
Building 30, Room 3300
1001 Potrero Avenue
San Francisco, CA 94110, USA

E-mail addresses:
sarah.goglin@ucsf.edu (S.E. Goglin)
John.Imboden@ucsf.edu (J.B. Imboden)

Primary Angiitis of the Central Nervous System

Jennifer Mandal, MD, Sharon A. Chung, MD, MAS*

KEYWORDS

- Primary angiitis of the central nervous system • Granulomatous angiitis of the CNS
- Amyloid beta-related angiitis • Neuroimaging • Brain biopsy
- Reversible cerebral vasoconstriction syndromes

KEY POINTS

- Primary angiitis of the central nervous system (PACNS) is rare and has a wide array of clinical presentations.
- PACNS presents a particularly daunting diagnostic challenge owing to the lack of reliable noninvasive diagnostic tests and the wide array of clinical mimics.
- Brain MRI is the most sensitive test for PACNS, with a normal MRI making PACNS very unlikely.
- Brain biopsy is neither highly sensitive nor specific for PACNS.
- Treatment of PACNS typically consists of either prednisone alone or the combination of prednisone and cyclophosphamide.

INTRODUCTION

Primary angiitis of the central nervous system (PACNS) is one of the most elusive and challenging diagnoses in all of rheumatology. PACNS, also called primary vasculitis of the CNS, refers to vasculitis that is confined to the brain, spinal cord, and meninges. The term *primary* is used to distinguish PACNS from *secondary* vasculitis of the CNS, in which the CNS manifestations are part of a systemic disease, such as infection, systemic vasculitis, connective tissue disease, or lymphoproliferative disorder.

Even for the most experienced clinicians, PACNS can present a perplexing and sometimes frustrating challenge. Owing to its broad and nonspecific array of possible clinical manifestations, PACNS is often included in the differential diagnosis for unusual or unexplained neurologic symptoms and yet, given its extreme rarity, PACNS is infrequently the correct diagnosis. This conundrum is further complicated by the

The authors have no disclosures and no conflicts of interest.
Division of Rheumatology, Russell/Engleman Rheumatology Research Center, University of California, San Francisco, 513 Parnassus Avenue, Medical Sciences S865, Box 0500, San Francisco, CA 94143-0500, USA
* Corresponding author.
E-mail address: sharon.chung@ucsf.edu

Rheum Dis Clin N Am 43 (2017) 503–518
http://dx.doi.org/10.1016/j.rdc.2017.06.001
0889-857X/17/© 2017 Elsevier Inc. All rights reserved.

rheumatic.theclinics.com

lack of a reliable noninvasive diagnostic test for PACNS, limited understanding of the etiopathogenesis of the disease, lack of controlled clinical trials or reliable animal models, and a wide array of clinical mimics (most notably the reversible cerebral vasoconstriction syndrome [RCVS]).

Despite the challenges posed by this rare and protean disease, our understanding of PACNS continues to improve as we develop a more nuanced awareness of the distinct subtypes of the disease, more reliable imaging and pathologic diagnostic tools, and a growing body of clinical research data from PACNS patient cohorts.

HISTORICAL CONTEXT

Some of the first case descriptions of PACNS were published in the 1950s by Newman and Wolf[1] and Cravioto and Feigin.[2] During the 1950s and through the 1970s, a few dozen case reports of PACNS were published, with nearly all of them diagnosing PACNS post mortem.[3] There was a dramatic increase in the number of case reports of PACNS in the 1980s as cerebral angiography became more accessible. Most of these cases lacked any pathologic confirmation. Many were treated with very aggressive immunosuppression regimens (typically cyclophosphamide [CYC] and high-dose glucocorticoids), owing to the common belief at the time that untreated PACNS was invariably fatal.[4] However, throughout the 1990s and early 2000s, a number of investigators realized that a sizable subset of patients diagnosed with PACNS based on angiography actually had a much more benign clinical course and favorable prognosis.[5,6] Over time, it became clear that many of these patients did not have true vasculitis, but rather a noninflammatory, reversible cerebral angiopathy.[7,8] The term reversible cerebral vasoconstriction syndrome (RCVS) was proposed by Calabrese and colleagues[7] in 2007, and this is now recognized as one of the most common and most important mimics of PACNS. RVCS is discussed in greater detail elsewhere in this article.

To facilitate understanding of this disease, PACNS patient cohorts have been established in France[9,10] and the United States (Mayo Clinic)[11,12]; each now contains more than 100 patients. In addition, an international cohort called The INTERnational Study on Primary Angiitis of the CEntral nervous system (INTERSPACE) was established in 2012.[13] From these cohorts, more detailed data have emerged regarding the clinical, radiographic, and pathologic characteristics of PACNS, as well as response to treatment.

EPIDEMIOLOGY

PACNS is extremely rare, accounting for only 1% of the systemic vasculitides, with an estimated annual incidence rate of 2.4 cases per 1,000,000 person-years, according to a retrospective analysis of a cohort of 163 cases.[12] There seems to be a male predominance of approximately 2:1, with a mean age of onset of approximately 50 years of age, although the disease can occur at virtually any age.[11,14,15]

CLINICAL MANIFESTATIONS

PACNS can present with a myriad of neurologic signs and symptoms, making both diagnosis and clinical research particularly challenging. Most patients with PACNS have a long prodromal period lasting several weeks to months (or in some cases, even years), during which the most common symptoms are headache and mild cognitive changes.[9,12] Sudden onset or a "thunderclap" headache is very rare in PACNS as opposed to in RCVS.[16] In a review of 116 reports of pathologically confirmed cases of PACNS, the mean time to diagnosis of PACNS from symptom onset was 170 days.[15]

After the prodromal period, patients with PACNS can present with a wide variety of neurologic manifestations (**Table 1**), including vision changes, cranial neuropathies, focal weakness, ataxia, stroke (typically multiple strokes in different vascular territories), and seizure.[9,11,12] Unlike most other vasculitides, constitutional symptoms such as fever, night sweats, and weight loss are relatively uncommon in PACNS.[11,12] Thus, prominent constitutional symptoms should raise the clinician's suspicion for an alternative diagnosis, such as a form of secondary CNS vasculitis.

Disease Subtypes

It is now increasingly recognized that PACNS is not a single entity, but rather an umbrella term for a number of distinct disease subtypes, affecting different parts of the CNS, different sized vessels, and with different histologic and pathologic findings on biopsy. A number of PACNS subtypes have been described, including granulomatous angiitis of the CNS (GACNS), lymphocytic angiitis of the CNS, amyloid beta-related angiitis, mass-like lesions, and spinal cord vasculitis.

Granulomatous Angiitis of the Central Nervous System

GACNS, although thought to be the most common subtype of PACNS, accounts for less than one-third of all cases of PACNS.[11,15] It typically presents with an insidious prodrome of headache or cognitive impairment or both, then progresses over 3 to 6 months to include focal neurologic deficits such as focal weakness, aphasia, ataxia, or seizure. Lumbar puncture is abnormal in approximately 90% of cases and has findings consistent with aseptic meningitis. Brain MRI typically shows scattered ischemic foci of varying ages, and cerebral angiography is normal in approximately 90% of cases because the disease affects primarily small vessels. Brain and leptomeningeal biopsies are necessary to confirm the diagnosis and to exclude mimics; histopathology demonstrates small to medium vessel vasculitis in the leptomeninges and cortex with granulomatous changes.[17] In an analysis of 136 GACNS cases, 51% of patients had an associated condition, including lymphoproliferative disorders, sarcoidosis, amyloidosis, or varicella zoster virus infection.[18]

Lymphocytic Angiitis of the Central Nervous System

The clinical presentation and neuroradiographic findings of lymphocytic angiitis of the CNS are very similar to GACNS, but lymphocytic angiitis of the CNS is distinguished by the presence of lymphocytic (instead of granulomatous) vasculitis on biopsy.[17]

Table 1
Clinical manifestations of PACNS at presentation

Characteristic	Mayo Cohort[12] (n = 163) (%)	French Cohort[9] (n = 52) (%)
Subacute or chronic headache	59.5	54
Cognitive impairment	54	35
Focal neurologic deficit or stroke	40.5	83
Aphasia	24.5	35
Seizure	20.2	33
Vision changes	37.4	15
Ataxia	19	12
Fever	9.8	13

Amyloid Beta-Related Angiitis

Cerebral amyloid angiopathy is characterized by beta-amyloid deposition in the vessels of the cerebral cortex and leptomeninges. Cerebral amyloid angiopathy, which affects approximately 30% to 50% of asymptomatic elderly patients and 80% of patients with Alzheimer's disease, is generally considered to be unrelated to PACNS. However, a small subset of patients with cerebral amyloid angiopathy develop a granulomatous, inflammatory CNS vasculitis, thought to be triggered by an immune response to amyloid beta. This entity, called amyloid beta-related angiitis is now considered a subtype of PACNS.[19–22] Patients with amyloid beta-related angiitis tend to be older at diagnosis (mean 65 years of age), have a higher prevalence of cognitive impairment (71%), and are more likely to have enhancement of leptomeningeal lesions on MRI.[21]

Mass-like Lesions

Approximately 5% of PACNS patients present with vasculitic mass lesions[23,24] (**Fig. 1**). These mass lesions can be indistinguishable from malignant tumors on MRI and angiography, and thus must be treated as suspected malignancies until proven otherwise via biopsy. Molloy and colleagues[23] reviewed 38 cases of PACNS presenting as mass-like lesions. The most common presenting symptoms were headache (74%), focal neurologic deficit (64%), diffuse neurologic deficit (50%), seizures (47%), and nausea and vomiting (21%). Unlike GACNS, which typically present with a long, indolent prodromal period, most patients with mass lesion PACNS presented within 1 month of symptom onset.

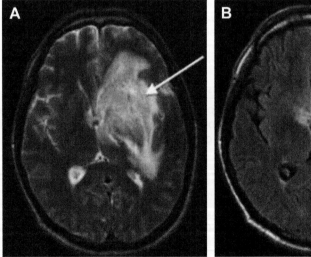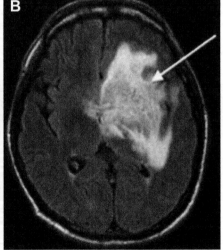

Fig. 1. Brain MRI of 51-year-old man with primary angiitis of the central nervous system (PACNS) presenting as a mass lesion. (*A*) Axial T2-weighted and (*B*) axial fluid-attenuated inversion recovery MRI demonstrating a large heterogeneous enhancing mass centered in the left basal ganglia (*arrow*). The appearance on MRI was initially suspicious for high-grade glioma or central nervous system lymphoma; however, a brain biopsy revealed PACNS. The patient responded well to treatment with prednisolone and intravenous cyclophosphamide. (*From* Gan C, Maingard J, Giles L, et al. Primary angiitis of the central nervous system presenting as a mass lesion. J Clin Neurosci 2015;22(9):1528–31.)

Spinal Cord Vasculitis

Spinal cord involvement is observed in approximately 5% of cases of PACNS,[24] but isolated spinal cord vasculitis (without concurrent brain involvement) is exceedingly rare and limited to a few case reports.[25–27] The thoracic spine is involved most commonly.[24]

DIAGNOSTIC APPROACH

Three diagnostic criteria for PACNS were proposed by Calabrese and Mallek in 1988.[3] Although our recognition of potential manifestations of PACNS has expanded, these 3 criteria can still indicate when to suspect PACNS:

1. History or clinical findings of an acquired neurologic deficit that remains unexplained after a thorough initial basic evaluation;
2. Either classic (high probability) angiographic evidence or histopathologic demonstration of angiitis within the CNS; and
3. No evidence of systemic vasculitis or any other condition to which the angiographic or pathologic condition could be attributed

Diagnosis of PACNS is challenging, owing to the lack of a single test with high sensitivity or specificity for PACNS, including brain biopsy, which is the gold standard.

Serologic Tests

There are no serologic tests with even moderate sensitivity or specificity for PACNS. Thus, the main value of serologic tests is to explore alternative diagnoses, such as infection, other systemic autoimmune diseases, or malignancy. Inflammatory markers such as erythrocyte sedimentation rate and C-reactive protein are typically normal in PACNS.[9,11,12] Extremely elevated erythrocyte sedimentation rate or C-reactive protein should heighten suspicion for a diagnosis other than PACNS.

Lumbar Puncture

Lumbar puncture should be performed in all patients with potential PACNS, unless there are strict contraindications. As with serologic testing, the primary value of evaluating cerebrospinal fluid (CSF) is to identify infectious or malignant causes. CSF evaluation shows at least 1 abnormal finding (all nonspecific) in 80% to 95% of patients with PACNS; completely normal CSF, therefore, argues against PACNS. The CSF abnormalities vary, but common findings include mild to moderate lymphocytic pleocytosis and/or elevated protein with normal glucose. More rarely, oligoclonal bands or elevated IgG can be seen.[11,12,28]

MRI

MRI should be performed on all patients with suspected PACNS. Recent case series report abnormal MRI findings in 95% to 100% of patients with PACNS,[12,16,29] reflecting the advances in MRI technique over the past decade. Thus, a normal brain MRI, particularly in combination with normal CSF analysis, is a very strong argument against a diagnosis of PACNS. The most common MRI findings in PACNS include multifocal infarcts, which are typically bilateral, distal, and across multiple vascular territories; leptomeningeal enhancement; and parenchymal enhancement[12,16,29] (**Fig. 2**). The frequency of parenchymal hemorrhage in PACNS varies widely in the recent literature, ranging from 8% in the Mayo cohort[12] to 55% in the French cohort.[29]

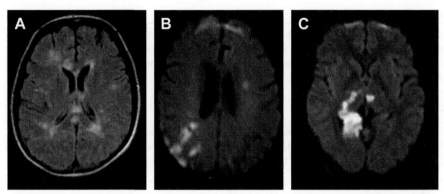

Fig. 2. MRI findings in primary angiitis of the central nervous system. (*A*) Multiple acute ischemic lesions in a 33-year-old man presenting with seizures and cognitive impairment. (*B*) Punctate acute infarcts in the left centrum semiovale in a 73-year-old woman presenting with vision loss. (*C*) Acute posterior circulation stroke in a 24-year-old man presenting with headache. (*Courtesy of* Grégoire Boulouis MD, MSc, Paris, France, and Olivier Naggara, MD, PhD, Paris, France.)

Magnetic Resonance Angiography and Computed Tomography Angiography

MR angiography (MRA) and computed tomography angiography (CTA) are less sensitive for PACNS than either MRI or conventional cerebral angiography. MRA and CTA are most useful for assessing large proximal arteries, whereas PACNS typically affects the small to medium vessels of the CNS. Narrowing of the large arteries on MRA or CTA should raise suspicion for an alternative process, such as RCVS, atherosclerosis, arterial dissection, fibromuscular dysplasia, or moyamoya disease. As MRA technology becomes more sophisticated (including high-resolution multicontrast wall and lumen imaging), its sensitivity for PACNS may improve,[30] and it may play a greater role in the evaluation of suspected PACNS.

Conventional Cerebral Angiography

Conventional angiography is frequently performed in cases where there is a high suspicion for PACNS. Compared with MRA and CTA, conventional angiography has better resolution for evaluating the medium vessels of the CNS. However, even digital subtraction angiography lacks the spatial resolution to evaluate the smallest vessels (<0.2 mm), limiting its sensitivity for PACNS to approximately 60% to 70%.[11,16,31,32] The angiographic findings of PACNS are nonspecific. Conventional angiography has an overall specificity estimated to be only 30%, in part because it cannot distinguish between vasculitis and vasculopathy. Findings may include alternating areas of vessel stenosis and dilatation, referred to as "beading," which is typically multifocal and bilateral. Less common findings include focal occlusions, collateral circulation, and, very rarely, microaneurysms, mass effect, delayed transit time, or cuffing. In 2016, Edgell and colleagues[32] proposed a modified grading system for cerebral angiographic findings in patients with suspected PACNS:

1. *High probability:* Vascular beading or alternating areas of stenosis and ectasia in multiple cerebral vessels.
2. *Medium probability:* Two or more low-frequency findings (focal occlusion, collateral circulation, microaneurysm, mass effect, delayed transit time, cuffing).
3. *Low probability:* A single low-frequency finding.

Brain Biopsy

Brain and leptomeningeal biopsy is considered the gold standard test for the diagnosis of PACNS and can also be critically important for ruling out mimics, such as infection and malignancy. A biopsy demonstrating vasculitis does not eliminate the need for careful tissue staining, culture, and cytology to evaluate thoroughly for causes of secondary vasculitis. In a review of 3 case series[33–35] of patients with a high pre-biopsy suspicion for PACNS based on clinical, CSF, and neuroimaging findings, brain biopsy revealed an alternative diagnosis in 35% of patients (46 of 132).[36]

A negative biopsy does not definitively rule out PACNS, because the false-negative rate may be as high as 25%.[4,37] This may be owing to sampling error, because PACNS can be patchy and spare large areas of the brain. Recommendations[38–42] have been made to increase the sensitivity of biopsy, including:

- The biopsy sample should be sufficiently large (at least 1 cm × 1 cm × 1 cm)
- The biopsy sample should contain leptomeninges, cortex, and subcortical white matter
- The biopsy site should be targeted from radiographically involved areas

The specific pathologic findings in PACNS vary based on the disease subtype, as discussed elsewhere in this article. In GACNS, pathologic findings include necrotizing vasculitis with poorly formed granulomas involving the small to medium vessels of the leptomeninges and cortex. In lymphocytic angiitis of the CNS, the inflammatory infiltrate is purely lymphocytic, without granulomas (**Fig. 3**). Amyloid beta-related angiitis is characterized by granulomatous vasculitis with beta amyloid deposition in the vessel walls. Other nonspecific pathologic findings are commonly observed on brain biopsy, including gliosis, mild perivascular mononuclear inflammation, and parenchymal infarct.[42,43]

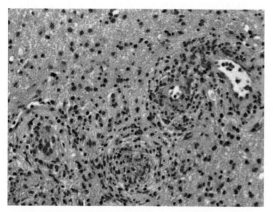

Fig. 3. Brain biopsy from a patient with lymphocytic angiitis of the central nervous system, demonstrating small blood vessels with a thickened intima and transmural involvement by a lymphohistiocytic inflammatory infiltrate, including focal fibrinoid necrosis (hematoxylin-eosin, 20×100). (*Courtesy of* Dr Arie Perry, and Dr Giselle Lopez San Francisco, CA.)

TREATMENT

There are no prospective studies examining treatment strategies in PACNS. The limited data available to guide treatment decisions are based on retrospective evaluation of patients with PACNS and extrapolation from other forms of systemic vasculitis. Treatment regimens often follow the paradigm established by antineutrophil cytoplasmic antibody–associated vasculitis—that is, more toxic medications are used for a short period of time to induce remission, followed by maintenance of remission with less toxic medications.

Remission Induction Therapy

Most patients with biopsy-proven PACNS are treated with immunosuppressive therapy. Several regimens have been described in the literature, and the 2 most common are either prednisone monotherapy or combination therapy with prednisone plus CYC.

In the Mayo cohort,[12] the largest PACNS cohort to date with 163 patients, 46% of patients were treated with prednisone monotherapy, and 44% were treated with prednisone plus CYC combination therapy. Across both groups, the median initial prednisone dose was 60 mg per day, and the average duration of prednisone therapy was 9 months. Patients treated with combination therapy tended to have more severe symptoms at presentation, with a higher frequency of stroke and higher Rankin disability scores, compared with those treated with prednisone alone. Favorable response to therapy was documented in 85% of the prednisone monotherapy group and 80% of the prednisone plus CYC group.[44] The overall mortality was 15% with a mean duration of follow-up of 12 months.

In comparison with the Mayo cohort, 82% of the patients in the French cohort[9] (52 patients), were treated with CYC plus glucocorticoid therapy. Patients in the French cohort also received a longer course of glucocorticoids (mean, 23 months). The mortality rate for this cohort was significantly lower, at 6%, with a mean duration of follow-up of 3 years, possibly owing to the increased use of combination therapy and longer duration of glucocorticoids.

Other induction regimens that have been described include prednisone plus azathioprine,[44] prednisone plus mycophenolate mofetil,[45,46] and prednisone plus rituximab.[47,48] There is currently insufficient evidence to adequately assess the efficacy of these regimens, although each may have efficacy based on the limited data available.

Remission Maintenance Therapy

Of the 97 patients followed by De Boysson and colleagues[10] in the French PACNS cohort (median followup of 4.5 years), 49% received remission maintenance therapy with a glucocorticoid-sparing agent. Azathioprine was used most commonly, with a few receiving either methotrexate or mycophenolate mofetil. Maintenance therapy was started on average 4 months after the initiation of glucocorticoid therapy. Patients who received maintenance therapy had a lower relapse rate (21%) compared with those who did not receive maintenance therapy (41%). Their data suggest a beneficial role for maintenance therapy (particularly azathioprine) in patients with PACNS who achieve remission after induction therapy. Fig. 4 illustrates a suggested approach to treatment of PACNS, based on data from the Mayo and French cohorts.

DIFFERENTIAL DIAGNOSIS

The differential diagnosis for PACNS is broad, and is summarized in Box 1. The majority of these diseases are discussed in detail in other articles of this issue. Herein we discuss 2 important mimics: RCVS and intravascular lymphoma (IVL).

Reversible Cerebral Vasoconstriction Syndrome

The most common angiographic mimic of PACNS is the RCVS. RCVS is a noninflammatory vasospastic syndrome associated with recurrent thunderclap headache, with

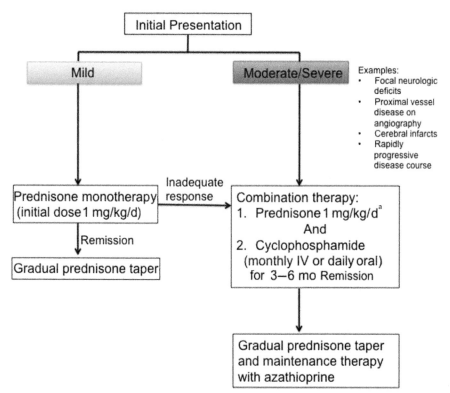

Fig. 4. A suggested approach to treatment of primary angiitis of the central nervous system.
[a] In severe cases, consider 3–5 days of pulse IV methylprednisolone first. IV, intravenous.

or without seizures and focal neurologic deficits. It occurs in the setting of diffuse vasoconstriction of the intracranial arteries that resolves within 3 months. RCVS has been reported in case series across different continents and racial and ethnic groups. Although the mean age of presentation is in the 5th decade of life (range, 42–45 years of age), both children and the elderly can be affected. A female predominance has been noted, with women being affected at least twice as common as men (female:-male 2–4:1).[16,49] Up to 60% of cases have been associated with an underlying condition or exposures, including pregnancy complications and vasoactive medication use (eg, pseudoephedrine, epinephrine, ergotamines).[50,51]

A key feature of RCVS is the recurrent thunderclap headache, which is seen on presentation in 90% to 95% of patients. Often described as "the worst headache of my life," this headache is severe and reaches peak intensity in less than 1 minute. It is often accompanied by nausea, vomiting, photophobia, and phonophobia. These headaches are typically bilateral, last 1 to 3 hours, and often recur over 1 to 4 weeks. Approximately 80% of patients are able to identify a trigger to the headache, such as stressful or emotional situations, Valsalva maneuvers, sexual activity, strenuous exercise, urinating, sneezing, coughing, laughing, or singing.[16,49,51] RCVS without the typical thunderclap headache has been described, but has not been well-reported. In this situation, RCVS is often diagnosed by angiography. Thus, the absence of a typical thunderclap headache does not exclude the diagnosis of RCVS.[52]

Other neurologic symptoms have also been observed. Seizures are reported in up to 20% of patients. Focal neurologic findings have been identified in up to 43% of

Box 1
Differential diagnosis for primary angiitis of the central nervous system

Infection

  Varicella zoster virus

  Cytomegalovirus

  Human immunodeficiency virus

  Neurosyphilis

  Tuberculosis

  Hepatitis B virus (associated with polyarteritis nodosa)

  Hepatitis C virus (associated with cryoglobulinemic vasculitis)

  Lyme disease

  Bartonella

  Fungi (*Aspergillus, Coccidiopdes, Histoplasma*)

  Cysticersosis

Malignancy

  Intravascular lymphoma

  Infiltrating glioma

  Carcinomatous meningitis

  Vasospastic disorders

  Reversible cerebral vasoconstriction syndrome

  Aneurysmal subarachnoid hemorrhage

  Pheochromocytoma

Systemic vasculitides and other rheumatologic diseases

  Antineutrophil cytoplasmic antibody–associated vasculitis

  Bechet's syndrome

  Polyarteritis nodosa

  Cryoglobulinemic vasculitis

  Systemic lupus erythematosus

  Sjögren syndrome

  Rheumatoid arthritis

  Antiphospholipid antibody syndrome

  Sarcoidosis

Other

  Cerebral emboli

  Atherosclerosis

  Cerebral artery dissection

  Moyamoya disease

  Fibromuscular dysplasia

  Radiation vasculopathy Neurofibromatosis

  Cerebral autosomal-dominant arteriopathy with subcortical infarcts and leukoencephalopathy

  Mitochondrial myopathy, encephalopathy, lactic acidosis, and strokelike episodes

patients, and include transient visual disturbances such as blurry vision, hemianopia, and scotomas. Persistent focal neurologic deficits include hemianopia and hemiplegia, and can occur owing to ischemic or hemorrhagic stroke.[50,51] Approximately 10% of patients experience permanent neurologic deficits.[7]

Diagnostic testing in RCVS is focused on differentiating RCVS from other causes of acute headache, including aneurysmal subarachnoid hemorrhage, sentinel bleed, cerebral venous sinus thrombosis, cervical artery dissection, and acute intracranial hypotension.[53] Urgent imaging with noncontrast computed tomography of the head is performed to exclude other causes of acute headache. The gold standard imaging study for diagnosis is digital subtraction angiography, which shows multifocal segmental vasoconstriction of the medium and large cerebral vessels ("sausage on a string"). However, given advancements in imaging techniques, other imaging modalities including CTA, MRI, and MRA, are also being used for diagnosis. Lumbar puncture should be performed if the head computed tomography is negative, and generally shows no or mild abnormalities, such as a mildly elevated lymphocyte count or mildly elevated protein levels. In RCVS, laboratory evaluations such as assessment of peripheral blood counts, renal function, liver enzymes, and inflammatory markers are usually normal. Brain biopsies are not recommended, unless the clinical presentation and diagnostic evaluation do not clearly support a diagnosis of RCVS or PACNS. To facilitate the diagnosis of RCVS, Calabrese and colleagues[7] proposed the following diagnostic criteria, with all 5 conditions needing to be met for a definite diagnosis of RCVS:

1. Acute and severe headache (often thunderclap), with or without neurologic deficits
2. Demonstration of multifocal segmental cerebral artery vasoconstriction via direct (catheter) or indirect angiography
3. Absence of aneurysmal subarachnoid hemorrhage
4. Normal, or near normal CSF analysis
5. Demonstration of reversibility of angiographic findings within 12 weeks of disease onset

To facilitate the differentiation between RCVS and PACNS, Singhal and colleagues[16] compared 159 RCVS patients with 47 patients with PACNS from a single institution. Clinical features differentiating RCVS from PACNS include thunderclap headache at onset (89% vs 6%; $P<.001$), recurrent thunderclap headache (85% vs 2%; $P<.001$), female gender (72% vs 28%; $P<.001$), and recent exposure to vasoconstrictive drugs (60% vs 28%; $P<.001$). Differences in initial imaging (computed tomography or MRI) features between RCVS and PACNS patients included the presence of infarcts (25% vs 81%; $P<.001$) and convexity subarachnoid hemorrhage (33% vs 2%; $P<.001$). When focusing on clinical, brain imaging, and CSF data to distinguish RCVS from PACNS, recurrent thunderclap headache had a 99% positive predictive value (53% negative predictive value) for RCVS. A single thunderclap headache was still highly predictive of RCVS (92% positive predictive value and 96% specificity), which increased to 100% with the addition of any one of these imaging findings: normal brain MRI, border zone–only infarcts, vasogenic edema, or fluid-attenuated inversion recovery sequence dot sign. In the absence of a thunderclap headache but with an abnormal cerebral angiogram, the presence of normal brain imaging, or vasogenic edema had 100% specificity and positive predictive value for RCVS, whereas the presence of deep gray or brainstem infarcts with an abnormal CSF had 100% specificity and positive predictive value for PACNS. Of note, this study only compared RCVS with PACNS, and thus these test performance characteristics may not be applicable if other diagnoses are also considered. **Table 2** presents clinical features that differ between patients with RCVS from PACNS.

Table 2
Clinical distinguishing features between RCVS and PACNS

Clinical Feature	RCVS	PACNS
Gender	Female predominant (2–4:1)	Male predominant
Onset	Acute, hours–days	Insidious, generally months
Clinical manifestations	Thunderclap headache in setting of trigger or associated condition	Chronic headaches with cognitive impairment
CSF analysis	Normal	Elevated WBC and/or protein
Initial CT or MRI	Abnormal in 70%	Abnormal in 100%
Cerebral angiography	Abnormal in 100%	Abnormal in 60%
Lobar hemorrhages	Common	Very rare
Convexity subarachnoid hemorrhage	Common	Very rare
Biopsy	No evidence of vasculitis (generally not performed)	Vasculitis seen in 60%–80%

Abbreviations: CSF, cerebrospinal fluid; CT, computed tomography; PACNS, primary angiitis of the central nervous system; RCVS, reversible cerebral vasoconstriction syndrome; WBC, white blood cell.

Adapted from Mehdi A, Hajj-Ali RA. Reversible cerebral vasoconstriction syndrome: a comprehensive update. Curr Pain Headache Rep 2014;18(9):443.

There are no randomized, controlled trials of the treatment for RCVS, and thus recommendations are based on observational cohort studies and expert opinion. Because most patients have a self-limited course, symptomatic headache management with analgesics and avoidance of triggers may be adequate to relieve symptoms and prevent reoccurrence. Although calcium channel blockers such as nimodipine, verapamil, and nicardipine have been used to reduce headaches, these agents have not been shown to alter the course of vasoconstriction or prevent neurologic deficits. Prednisone use is not recommended and may be associated with worse functional outcomes.[54] Neurovascular interventions such as balloon angioplasty and intra-arterial administration of vasodilators such as milrinone and nimodipine have been used with mixed results, and thus are reserved for severe, refractory cases.[50,51]

Intravascular Lymphoma

Another mimic of PACNS is IVL, which is differentiated from PACNS by tissue biopsy. IVL is a rare type of non-Hodgkin's lymphoma that is characterized by the growth of neoplastic lymphocytes within the lumen of predominately small and medium sized blood vessels. This cell proliferation within the vessels may block blood flow to downstream tissues, resulting in tissue ischemia.[55]

IVL typically affects older patients, with more than 70% of patients diagnosed after the age of 60. Geographic differences in clinical manifestations have been observed. In patients from Western countries, CNS (34%–52%) and cutaneous manifestations (24%–39%) are most common. Skin manifestations are varied, and include painful erythematous induration, violaceous plaques, cellulitis, ulcerated nodules, and generalized telangiectasia. In contrast, patients from Asian countries have a lesser prevalence of neurologic manifestations (25%) with a greater prevalence of fever (74%) and hematologic abnormalities such has hemophagocytosis (59%) and thrombocytopenia (58%–76%).[55,56] IVL is considered a disseminated disease at diagnosis and can involve other organ systems including the kidneys, liver, and lungs.

In a meta-analysis of 654 patients with IVL,[57] neurologic manifestations were observed in 338 patients (52%). Of the 276 patients (42%) with CNS involvement, cognitive impairment or dementia were the most commonly observed at presentation, affecting 61% of patients. Other neurologic manifestations seen on presentation include paralysis and paraplegia (22%), seizures (13.4%), visual disturbances (8.7%), ataxia (7.6%), and strokelike symptoms (7.6%). Patients often have more than 1 neurologic manifestation on presentation.[55]

Neuroimaging findings of IVL can be nonspecific and can resemble findings seen in PACNS. Although MRI can show nonspecific hyperintensities of the white matter suggesting small vessel ischemic disease or demyelination, abnormalities are observed in one-half of patients with neurologic manifestations.[55] Abnormalities in blood counts are often seen, including anemia (63%–78%) and increased serum lactate dehydrogenase and β2-microglobulin levels (>80%).[56] Diagnosis relies on biopsy of involved tissue demonstrating neoplastic lymphocytes in the small and medium vessels, such as the capillaries and postcapillary venules. Of note, random deep skin biopsies that contain subcutaneous tissue can be diagnostic, even in Asian populations where cutaneous involvement is less common.[55] It is important to recognize that neoplastic proliferation of lymphocytes can occur in other lymphoproliferative disorders, and large lymphoid cells can be found intravascularly in nonneoplastic conditions such as infectious mononucleosis.[56]

SUMMARY

PACNS presents a particularly daunting diagnostic and treatment challenge, owing its wide array of nonspecific clinical manifestations, the lack of any highly specific diagnostic test, and the absence of prospective research data. Although it is important to consider PACNS in the differential diagnosis for patients with unexplained neurologic symptoms or neuroimaging findings, the clinician must always maintain a high degree of skepticism, and search thoroughly for other potential culprits within the long list of PACNS mimics. As new data continue to emerge from the PACNS patient cohorts, we will continue to refine and enhance our understanding of this rare disease.

REFERENCES

1. Newman W, Wolf A. Non-infectious granulomatous angiitis involving the central nervous system. Trans Am Neurol Assoc 1952;56:114–7.
2. Cravioto H, Feigin I. Granulomatous angiitis of the central nervous system. Neurology 1959;9:599–609.
3. Calabrese LH, Mallek JA. Primary angiitis of the central nervous system: report of 8 new cases, review of the literature, and proposal for diagnostic criteria. Medicine 1988;67(1):20.
4. Cupps TR, Moore PM, Fauci AS. Isolated angiitis of the central nervous system. Am J Med 1983;74(1):97–105.
5. Call GK, Fleming MC, Sealfon S, et al. Reversible cerebral segmental vasoconstriction. Stroke 1988;19(9):1159–70.
6. Calabrese LH, Cragg LA, Furlan AJ. Benign angiopathy: a distinct subset of angiographically defined primary angiitis of the central nervous system. J Rheumatol 1993;20(12):2046–50.
7. Calabrese LH, Dodick DW, Schwedt TJ, et al. Narrative review: reversible cerebral vasoconstriction syndromes. Ann Intern Med 2007;146(1):34–44.

8. Singhal AB. Postpartum angiopathy with reversible posterior leukoencephalopathy. Arch Neurol 2004;61(3):411–6.
9. Boysson H, Zuber M, Naggara O, et al. Primary angiitis of the central nervous system: description of the first fifty-two adults enrolled in the French cohort of patients with primary vasculitis of the central nervous system. Arthritis Rheumatol 2014;66(5):1315–26.
10. de Boysson H, Parienti J-J, Arquizan C, et al. Maintenance therapy is associated with better long-term outcomes in adult patients with primary angiitis of the central nervous system. Rheumatology (Oxford) 2017. [Epub ahead of print].
11. Salvarani C, Brown RD, Calamia KT, et al. Primary central nervous system vasculitis: analysis of 101 patients. Ann Neurol 2007;62(5):442–51.
12. Salvarani C, Brown RD Jr, Christianson T, et al. An update of the mayo clinic cohort of patients with adult primary central nervous system vasculitis: description of 163 patients. Medicine 2015;94(21):e738.
13. Lanthier S, Calabrese LH, Ferro JM, et al. The INTERnational Study on Primary Angiitis of the CEntral nervous system – a call to the world. Int J Stroke 2014; 9(5):E23.
14. Calabrese LH. Vasculitis of the central nervous system. Rheum Dis Clin North Am 1995;21(4):1059–76.
15. Calabrese LH, Duna GF, Lie JT. Vasculitis in the central nervous system. Arthritis Rheumatol 1997;40(7):1189–201.
16. Singhal AB, Topcuoglu MA, Fok JW, et al. Reversible cerebral vasoconstriction syndromes and primary angiitis of the central nervous system: clinical, imaging, and angiographic comparison. Ann Neurol 2016;79(6):882–94.
17. Suri V, Kakkar A, Sharma MC, et al. Primary angiitis of the central nervous system: a study of histopathological patterns and review of the literature. Folia Neuropathol 2014;52(2):187–96.
18. Younger DS, Kass RM. Vasculitis and the nervous system. Neurol Clin 1997;15(4): 737–58.
19. Scolding NJ, Joseph F, Kirby PA, et al. Aβ-related angiitis: primary angiitis of the central nervous system associated with cerebral amyloid angiopathy. Brain 2005; 128(3):500–15.
20. Rigby H, Easton A, Bhan V. Amyloid β-related angiitis of the central nervous system: report of 3 cases. Can J Neurol Sci 2011;38(4):626–30.
21. Danve A, Grafe M, Deodhar A. Amyloid beta-related angiitis—a case report and comprehensive review of literature of 94 cases. Semin Arthritis Rheum 2014; 44(1):86–92.
22. Nouh A, Borys E, Gierut AK, et al. Amyloid-beta related angiitis of the central nervous system: case report and topic review. Front Neurol 2014;5:13.
23. Molloy ES, Singhal AB, Calabrese LH. Tumour-like mass lesion: an under-recognised presentation of primary angiitis of the central nervous system. Ann Rheum Dis 2008;67(12):1732–5.
24. Salvarani C, Brown RD, Calamia KT, et al. Primary CNS vasculitis with spinal cord involvement. Neurology 2008;70(24 Pt 2):2394–400.
25. Campi A, Benndorf G, Martinelli V, et al. Spinal cord involvement in primary angiitis of the central nervous system: a report of two cases. Am J Neuroradiol 2001; 22(3):577–82.
26. Goertz C, Wegner C, Brück W, et al. Primary angiitis of the CNS with pure spinal cord involvement: a case report. J Neurol 2010;257(10):1762–4.
27. Ropper AH, Ayata C, Adelman L. Vasculitis of the spinal cord. Arch Neurol 2003; 60(12):1791–4.

28. Hajj-Ali RA, Furlan A, Abou-Chebel A, et al. Benign angiopathy of the central nervous system: cohort of 16 patients with clinical course and long-term followup. Arthritis Rheum 2002;47(6):662–9.

29. Boulouis G, de Boysson H, Zuber M, et al. Primary angiitis of the central nervous system: magnetic resonance imaging spectrum of parenchymal, meningeal, and vascular lesions at baseline. Stroke 2017;48(5):1248–55.

30. Cosottini M, Canovetti S, Pesaresi I, et al. 3-T magnetic resonance angiography in primary angiitis of the central nervous system. J Comput Assist Tomogr 2013; 37(4):493–8.

31. Vollmer TL, Guarnaccia J, Harrington W, et al. Idiopathic granulomatous angiitis of the central nervous system. Diagnostic challenges. Arch Neurol 1993;50(9): 925–30.

32. Edgell RC, Sarhan AE, Soomro J, et al. The role of catheter angiography in the diagnosis of central nervous system vasculitis. Interv Neurol 2016;5(3–4): 194–208.

33. Alrawi A, Trobe JD, Blaivas M, et al. Brain biopsy in primary angiitis of the central nervous system. Neurology 1999;53(4):858–60.

34. Castle J, Llinas R, Wityk R. Biopsy proven isolated CNS vasculitis, much-vaunted but rarely seen: 20 year retrospective review of brain biopsies. Stroke 2008;39:574.

35. Chu CT, Gray L, Goldstein LB. Diagnosis of intracranial vasculitis: a multidisciplinary approach. J Neuropathol Exp Neurol 1998;57(1):30–8.

36. Powers WJ. Primary angiitis of the central nervous system: diagnostic criteria. Neurol Clin 2015;33(2):515–26.

37. Calabrese LH, Furlan AJ, Gragg LA, et al. Primary angiitis of the central nervous system: diagnostic criteria and clinical approach. Cleve Clin J Med 1992;59(3): 293–306.

38. Hajj-Ali RA, Singhal AB, Benseler S, et al. Primary angiitis of the CNS. Lancet Neurol 2011;10(6):561–72.

39. Lanthier S. Primary angiitis of the central nervous system in children: 10 cases proven by biopsy. J Rheumatol 2002;29(7):1575–6.

40. Hurst RW, Grossman RI. Neuroradiology of central nervous system vasculitis. Semin Neurol 1994;14(4):320–40.

41. Salvarani C, Brown RD, Calamia KT, et al. Angiography-negative primary central nervous system vasculitis: a syndrome involving small cerebral vessels. Medicine 2008;87(5):264–71.

42. Miller DV, Salvarani C, Hunder GG, et al. Biopsy findings in primary angiitis of the central nervous system. Am J Surg Pathol 2009;33(1):35–43.

43. Giannini C, Salvarani C, Hunder G, et al. Primary central nervous system vasculitis: pathology and mechanisms. Acta Neuropathol 2012;123(6):759–72.

44. Salvarani C, Brown RD, Christianson TJH, et al. Adult primary central nervous system vasculitis treatment and course: analysis of one hundred sixty-three patients. Arthritis Rheumatol 2015;67(6):1637–45.

45. Rosati A, Cosi A, Basile M, et al. Mycophenolate mofetil as induction and long-term maintaining treatment in childhood: primary angiitis of the central nervous system. Joint Bone Spine 2016;84(3):353–6.

46. Salvarani C, Brown RD, Christianson TJH, et al. Mycophenolate mofetil in primary central nervous system vasculitis. Semin Arthritis Rheum 2015;45(1):55–9.

47. Salvarani C, Brown RD, Huston J, et al. Treatment of primary CNS vasculitis with rituximab: case report. Neurology 2014;82(14):1287–8.

48. de Boysson H, Arquizan C, Guillevin L, et al. Rituximab for primary angiitis of the central nervous system: report of 2 patients from the French COVAC cohort and review of the literature. J Rheumatol 2013;40(12):2102–3.
49. Ducros A, Wolff V. The typical thunderclap headache of reversible cerebral vasoconstriction syndrome and its various triggers. Headache 2016;56(4):657–73.
50. Cappelen-Smith C, Calic Z, Cordato D. Reversible cerebral vasoconstriction syndrome: recognition and treatment. Curr Treat Options Neurol 2017;19(6):21.
51. Mehdi A, Hajj-Ali RA. Reversible cerebral vasoconstriction syndrome: a comprehensive update. Curr Pain Headache Rep 2014;18(9):443.
52. Wolff V, Ducros A. Reversible cerebral vasoconstriction syndrome without typical thunderclap headache. Headache 2016;56(4):674–87.
53. Schwedt TJ, Matharu MS, Dodick DW. Thunderclap headache. Lancet Neurol 2006;5(7):621–31.
54. Singhal AB, Topcuoglu MA. Glucocorticoid-associated worsening in reversible cerebral vasoconstriction syndrome. Neurology 2017;88(3):228–36.
55. Shimada K, Kinoshita T, Naoe T, et al. Presentation and management of intravascular large B-cell lymphoma. Lancet Oncol 2009;10(9):895–902.
56. Ponzoni M, Ferreri AJM, Campo E, et al. Definition, diagnosis, and management of intravascular large B-cell lymphoma: proposals and perspectives from an international consensus meeting. Am Soc Clin Oncol 2007;25:3168–73.
57. Fonkem E, Dayawansa S, Stroberg E, et al. Neurological presentations of intravascular lymphoma (IVL): meta-analysis of 654 patients. BMC Neurol 2016; 16(1):9.

Neurologic Manifestations of Primary Sjögren Syndrome

 CrossMark

Mary Margaretten, MD, MAS

KEYWORDS

- Primary Sjögren syndrome • Peripheral neuropathy • Central nervous system

KEY POINTS

- Patients with primary Sjögren syndrome may exhibit a variety of peripheral neuropathies or central nervous system (CNS) manifestations.
- The underlying mechanisms in the pathogenesis of CNS involvement in primary Sjögren syndrome seem to be immune-mediated vasculopathy, vasculitis, or demyelination.
- The heterogeneity of neurologic manifestations in primary Sjögren syndrome complicates the approach to treatment, which should be directed toward the underlying neuropathologic mechanism.

Primary Sjögren syndrome is an autoimmune inflammatory disease characterized by mononuclear lymphocytic infiltration of exocrine (ie, salivary and lacrimal) glands in the setting of antinuclear antibodies, particularly to Ro/SSA and La/SSB, and that occurs in the absence of another autoimmune disease. Patients with primary Sjögren syndrome can develop extraglandular manifestations, such as joint, muscle, pulmonary, kidney, and skin involvement.[1] Neurologic manifestations of primary Sjögren syndrome range in prevalence from 8% to 49%. The true prevalence of neurologic manifestation in primary Sjögren syndrome is likely in the middle range of these estimates and most studies suggest a prevalence of 20%.[2–6] The wide range of reported frequency is due to (1) the evolving classification criteria of primary Sjögren syndrome,[7–9] (2) whether neurologic manifestations are clinically apparent versus asymptomatic, that is, neuropathies detected by a neurologist using electrophysiologic studies[10] or nonspecific white matter changes seen on brain MRI,[11] (3) the heterogeneity of neurologic manifestations ranging from multiple sclerosis (MS)–like central nervous system (CNS) involvement[12] to entrapment neuropathies like carpal tunnel syndrome[13] to psychiatric disorders[14] such as depression,[15–17] and (4) selection bias of patients on the basis of a primary neurologic diagnosis.

Disclosures: None.
Division of Rheumatology, University of California San Francisco, 1001 Potrero Street, Building 30, San Francisco, CA 94110, USA
E-mail address: Mary.margaretten@ucsf.edu

Rheum Dis Clin N Am 43 (2017) 519–529
http://dx.doi.org/10.1016/j.rdc.2017.06.002
0889-857X/17/© 2017 Elsevier Inc. All rights reserved.

rheumatic.theclinics.com

PERIPHERAL NEUROPATHY

Patients with primary Sjögren syndrome may exhibit a variety of peripheral neuropathies (**Table 1**). Distal sensory and sensorimotor neuropathies are the most common manifestations of peripheral nerve disease in primary Sjögren syndrome. Sensory neuropathies include painful nonataxic sensory polyneuropathy, dorsal root ganglionitis, and trigeminal neuropathy. Patients with primary Sjögren syndrome can suffer from severe neuropathic pain with small fiber neuropathy causing lancinating or burning pain that is length or not length dependent. The pain can affect the proximal torso, extremities, and/or the face. Subtypes of sensorimotor neuropathies are sensorimotor polyneuropathy and mononeuritis multiplex. Other forms of peripheral neuropathies, more rarely associated with primary Sjögren syndrome, are polyradiculoneuritis, autonomic neuropathy, or motor neuron disorder.[18] All these peripheral neuropathies can be differentiated according to clinical presentation and results from electromyography and nerve-conduction studies, evoked potentials, and nerve and muscle biopsy. Skin biopsy may provide useful information to diagnose small fiber neuropathies by assessing for the intraepidermal nerve fiber density of unmyelinated nerves, especially when there is a non–length-dependent distribution. A rational approach to diagnosis and treatment requires a careful appraisal of the clinical subtype of the peripheral neuropathy, as well as a familiarity with the pathophysiologic mechanisms.

The pathogenesis of peripheral neuropathies is varied and depends on the type of nerve involved. Pathology in cases of sensory ganglioneuronopathy consists of loss of neuronal cell bodies and lymphocytic infiltration. Similarly, ganglionitis is caused by lymphocytic infiltration into the dorsal root ganglia with or without accompanying vasculitis.[19] Conversely, vasculitis has been implicated as the main mechanism of disease in other peripheral neuropathies, such as mononeuritis multiplex. A review of 33 patients with primary Sjögren syndrome at the Mayo Clinic with 11 sural nerve biopsies revealed perivascular inflammatory infiltrates and other vessel abnormalities, which were diagnostic in 2 cases and strongly suggestive of necrotizing vasculitis in 6 cases. The vascular or perivascular inflammation occurs in the small epineurial vessels, both the arterioles and venules. Axonal degeneration predominates over demyelination and is focal or multifocal. Loss of myelinated nerve fibers is common and loss of small diameter nerve fibers occurs.[20]

Painful Sensory Neuropathy

This is a small fiber neuropathy that presents with painful dysesthesias in the most distal portions of the limbs, usually beginning in the lower extremities, for example, "burning feet." In the majority of patients, the spread of dysesthesias is chronic, occurring over months to years. Affected patients most commonly have a distal and symmetric distribution of burning paresthesia, most likely owing to an axonopathy.[21] Painful sensory neuropathies in primary Sjögren syndrome typically have no electrophysiologic findings, unless there is a concomitant large fiber neuropathy.[22]

"Pure" Small Fiber Dorsal Root Ganglionitis

Some patients have painful dysesthesias in an asymmetric, patchy, non–length-dependent distribution. This may represent a dorsal root ganglionitis affecting small neurons. Pathology in cases of sensory ganglioneuronopathy consists of loss of neuronal cell bodies and lymphocytic infiltration with clustering around neurons.[23]

Table 1
Types of peripheral neuropathies in primary Sjögren syndrome

Peripheral Neuropathy	Clinical Manifestations	Diagnostic Study Results (MRI, Nerve Conduction Study, Nerve Biopsy)
Sensory neuropathy		
Painful sensory neuropathy	Painful dysesthesias in the most distal portions of the limbs, usually the lower extremities that is, "burning feet"	Usually no electrophysiologic findings unless there is a concomitant large fiber neuropathy
"Pure" dorsal root ganglionitis	Painful, asymmetric, patchy dysesthesias in a non–length-dependent distribution	Small fiber involvement only, CD8+ lymphocytic infiltration with clustering around neurons
"Mixed" dorsal root ganglionitis[a]	Areflexia, autonomic instability (Adie's pupil, tachycardia, anhidrosis, orthostatic hypotension)	High-intensity signal on T2-weighted MRI of the dorsal columns of the spinal cord. Small and large fiber involvement and CD8+ lymphocytic infiltration with clustering around neurons
Sensorimotor neuropathy		
Sensorimotor polyneuropathy	Parasthesias and distal symmetric muscle weakness (toe or foot extensors); reflexes may be diminished or absent	Nerve conduction studies with axonal polyneuropathy affecting motor and sensory fibers
Mononeuritis multiplex	Nerve damage in 2 or more named nerves in separate parts of the body, that is, wrist drop caused by infarction of the radial nerve and foot drop caused by damage to the peroneal nerve	Specific for the diagnosis of vasculitic neuropathy
Cranial neuropathies		
Trigeminal neuropathy	Paroxysmal attacks of sharp, or stabbing pain in the distribution of branches of the fifth cranial nerve	
Cranial nerves	VII (Bell palsy), VII (neural deafness and vestibular dysfunction), III, IV, or VI (diplopia)	
Radiculoneuropathy	Progressive sensory impairment and muscle weakness	Cerebrospinal fluid protein concentration is usually elevated, but pleocytosis is absent
Autonomic neuropathy	Delayed gastric emptying, orthostatic hypotension, hypohidrosis or anhidrosis, bladder dysfunction, constipation, Adie's pupils	Tilt table test

[a] Also known as sensory ataxic neuropathy.

"Mixed" Small and Large Fiber Dorsal Root Ganglionitis

This rare sensory ataxic neuropathy is characterized by the prominent loss of kinesthesia and proprioception, leading to gait ataxia. Generalized areflexia is typically present. Autonomic lesions occur, including Adie's pupil (a dilated pupil that is poorly reactive to light but does react slowly to accommodation), fixed tachycardia, anhidrosis, and orthostatic hypotension. Patients with advanced disease may become wheelchair bound. High-intensity signal is often demonstrated on T2-weighted MRI of the dorsal columns of the spinal cord.[24] As with a pure small fiber dorsal root ganglionitis, this neuropathy is a dorsal root ganglionitis with CD8[+] lymphocytic infiltration clustering around neurons.[23]

Sensorimotor Polyneuropathy

Patients with this type of neuropathy may initially complain of distal paresthesias and exhibit sensory deficits similar to those with sensory neuropathy. The sensory symptoms, however, are gradually accompanied by muscle weakness in a distal, symmetric distribution. The weakness is usually mild and limited to the toe or foot extensors, but rare severe cases may require assistance of a cane for ambulation. Deep tendon reflexes may be diminished or absent. Nerve conduction studies typically reveal an axonal polyneuropathy affecting motor and sensory fibers. Nerve biopsy is not recommended, unless the presence of vasculitis is suspected. Extraglandular disease is more frequent and more severe, compared with patients with sensory polyneuropathy and often accompanied by palpable purpura, vasculitis, low C4 complement factor, and cryoglobulinemia.[25] There is an association between primary Sjögren syndrome, sensorimotor polyneuropathy, cryoglobulinemia, and the development of lymphoma.[26]

Mononeuritis Multiplex

Mononeuritis multiplex encompasses the vasculitic neuropathies, and, although rare in primary Sjögren syndrome, when promptly diagnosed and treated, mononeuritis multiplex may be the peripheral nerve manifestation that exhibits the most dramatic and durable response to therapy.[27] Because the longest nerves in the body are affected first, foot drop is the most common manifestation of mononeuritis multiplex. Patients are often unaware of dorsiflexion weakness; patients with tibialis anterior weakness must raise their knee on the affected side high to avoid tripping over the weakened foot, leading to a "foot-slapping" gait. Nerve infarction eventually leads to muscle wasting, which, in many cases, is permanent. There is decreased survival in patients with primary Sjögren syndrome with peripheral neuropathy, especially in those with mononeuritis multiplex and sensorimotor polyneuropathy, in comparison to patients with primary Sjögren syndrome without peripheral neuropathy.[28] Nerve and muscle biopsy may be required to confirm the diagnosis of vasculitic neuropathy unless vasculitis is confirmed by biopsy of other involved organs. Biopsy of affected nerves often shows axonal degeneration and a perivascular inflammatory infiltrate, suggesting an underlying vasculitis cause in many cases. Patients with primary Sjögren syndrome mononeuritis multiplex should be evaluated for underlying cryoglobulinemia.

Cranial Neuropathies

Cranial mononeuropathies and polyneuropathies have been reported in primary Sjögren syndrome.[29] The most common cranial neuropathy is a trigeminal neuropathy. The trigeminal nerve provides sensation for the face and the motor supply to the muscles of mastication. It has 3 major divisions: ophthalmic, maxillary, and mandibular. Trigeminal nerve dysfunction in primary Sjögren syndrome is caused by damage to the ganglion.[30] The ophthalmic division is usually spared, thereby preserving the corneal reflex. Other cranial nerves affected in primary Sjögren syndrome are VII (Bell palsy), VIII (resulting in neural deafness and vestibular dysfunction), and III, IV, or VI (resulting in diplopia). Hearing may also be affected in a significant proportion of patients, although many cases are subclinical.[31,32]

Radiculoneuropathy

This rare disorder is characterized by sensorimotor dysfunction with both progressive sensory impairment and muscle weakness. The primary lesion in these patients seems to be in the spinal nerve roots or in the most proximal nerve trunks, consistent with an inflammatory radiculoneuropathy. The cerebrospinal fluid protein concentration is usually increased , but pleocytosis is absent.

Autonomic Neuropathy

The prevalence of autonomic neuropathy is difficult to estimate,[25] but mild autonomic dysfunction occurs in primary Sjögren syndrome as evidenced by abnormal cardiovascular reflex testing,[33] delayed gastric emptying,[34] and bladder dysfunction. Clinically overt autonomic neuropathies are manifested by severe orthostatic hypotension, hypohidrosis or anhidrosis of the trunk and limbs, abdominal pain, constipation, diarrhea, and Adie's pupils.[35,36] Features of autonomic dysfunction can occur in conjunction with other sensory neuropathies. One study shows that patients with primary Sjögren syndrome who had sensory or motor peripheral neuropathies, additionally 57% had Adie's pupils, 40% had orthostatic hypotension, and 70% had abnormal sweating.[3]

CENTRAL NERVOUS SYSTEM

The CNS consists of the brain and spinal cord, of which any part may be affected by primary Sjögren syndrome. CNS manifestations associated with primary Sjögren syndrome are varied and the clinical spectrum encompass focal central lesions, conditions that mimic MS,[37] encephalitis,[38] aseptic meningitis,[39] cerebellar syndromes causing ataxia,[40–42] movement disorders affecting the basal ganglia producing chorea,[43,44] neuromyelitis optica,[4,45] and problems with memory,[46] cognition,[16,47] and depression. CNS involvement frequently precedes the diagnosis of primary Sjögren syndrome and often transpires as recurrent, multifocal episodes separated by long disease-free intervals resulting in insidious progressive neurologic deficits.[2] Similar to peripheral neuropathies, the frequency of CNS involvement in primary Sjögren syndrome is imprecise and estimates vary widely. Lung involvement, disease duration, and decreased C4 in primary Sjögren syndrome are predictors for CNS involvement.[4]

The underlying mechanisms in the pathogenesis of CNS involvement in primary Sjögren syndrome seem to be immunologically mediated small vessel vasculopathy and, less often, a true small vessel vasculitis.[48] Evidence to support this hypothesis of immunologically mediated vasculopathy and vasculitis being the drivers of CNS disease in primary Sjögren syndrome includes (1) the cerebrospinal fluid of patients with primary Sjögren syndrome and active CNS disease can show lymphocytosis, an increased IgG index, increased protein level, and/or oligoclonal bands on electrophoresis,[2,39,49,50] (2) evidence of intrathecal activation of the terminal pathway of complement in 1 study of cerebrospinal fluid from patients with primary Sjögren syndrome and CNS involvement,[51] (3) histopathology from brain tissue in some patients with primary Sjögren syndrome demonstrates a small vessel lymphocytic inflammatory and ischemic vasculopathy,[35] (4) concomitant active peripheral vasculitis affecting the skin, muscles, and nerves occurs in up to 75% of patients with primary Sjögren syndrome and active CNS disease,[52] and (5) small vessel vasculitis is found in a significant proportion of patients with primary Sjögren syndrome CNS undergoing cerebral angiography. In these patients, there was a strong correlation between abnormal angiography findings and anti–SS-A/Ro antibody positivity.[53]

The usefulness of MRI in characterizing CNS involvement in primary Sjögren syndrome is unclear. Nonspecific T2-weighted hyperintensity occurs in most patients with focal CNS involvement,[54] but is less likely to pick up pathologies in diffuse CNS disease. However, the findings for the former are not specific for CNS disease in primary Sjögren syndrome. Frontal white matter microstructure alterations on MRI have been found to be associated clinically with mild cognitive impairment in some studies,[55] but the interpretation of this association is hampered by the lack of a standard with which to interpret these MRI findings and by the difficulties in distinguishing MRI abnormalities owing to primary Sjögren syndrome from similar abnormalities owing to age and cerebrovascular disease.[56]

Subacute Encephalopathy

Diffuse manifestations of CNS involvement in primary Sjögren syndrome may present as subacute encephalitis, often occurring as acute episodes, with memory loss, cognitive dysfunction, visual disturbances, and dizziness.[2,4] Often, aseptic meningitis, cognitive dysfunction with dementia, and psychiatric abnormalities are lumped into this "diffuse" category of CNS involvement with primary Sjögren syndrome.

Multiple Sclerosis–like Disease

Patients with clearly diagnosed primary Sjögren syndrome can develop MS-like CNS involvement characterized by a relapsing–remitting course with neurologic episodes distributed in space and time. Concomitant optic neuritis may be observed and brain MRI can show multiple diffuse subcortical and periventricular white matter lesions. cerebrospinal fluid analysis may demonstrate a lymphocyte pleocytosis and detection of oligoclonal bands.[4] MS-like syndromes could represent a subset of neuro-Sjogren's disease although a population-based study did not find an increased association of MS with primary Sjögren syndrome,[15] so the high frequency found in retrospective cross-sectional case-control studies may be due to selection bias, which can lead to overestimation of this MS-like syndrome in primary Sjögren syndrome.

Headache

Although a link between migraine headaches and primary Sjögren syndrome has been studied, with Raynaud's phenomenon as the suggested mechanism,[57] migraines and headache are not more common in patients with primary Sjögren syndrome compared with healthy individuals.[58]

Psychiatric Disease

Primary Sjögren syndrome does increase the risk of comorbid psychiatric disorders, such as depression, anxiety, and sleep disorders.[14] Given that patients with chronic diseases are at higher risk for depression, anxiety, and sleep disorders,[59,60] it is unclear whether primary Sjögren syndrome confers an independent increased risk of psychiatric disease.[61]

Ischemic Stroke

Although accelerated atherosclerosis is seen in patients with inflammatory, autoimmune conditions such as systemic vasculitis, rheumatoid arthritis, and systemic lupus erythematous, this is not the case with primary Sjögren syndrome. A retrospective cohort study involving more than 4000 patients with primary Sjögren syndrome did not find an increased risk of ischemic stroke compared with age-, gender-, and comorbidity-matched controls.[62] However, antiphospholipid antibodies and lupus anticoagulants are more frequent in patients with primary Sjögren syndrome and, if present, contribute to an increased risk of central thromboembolic events.[63]

MYOPATHY

Occasionally, patients with primary Sjögren syndrome present with weakness, and, in this cyclical scenario, an inflammatory myopathy should be considered either as an overlap syndrome with another rheumatic disease or as an inflammatory myopathy of primary Sjögren syndrome.[64] There are case reports of patients with primary Sjögren syndrome presenting with quadriparesis, but this is not a neurologic manifestation of primary Sjögren syndrome, but rather a metabolic issue of hypokalemic quadriparesis.[65–67]

Treatment

Clinically significant neurologic manifestations in patients with primary Sjögren syndrome may warrant aggressive therapy with glucocorticoids and immunosuppressive agents. Unfortunately, there are no randomized controlled trials evaluating intravenous immunoglobulin and/or immunosuppressive medications in patients with primary Sjögren syndrome and neuropathies or CNS disease. Recommendations are based on limited evidence of small, uncontrolled series[68] and often treatment for the neurologic manifestations of primary Sjögren syndrome is extrapolated from treatment of other organ systems in primary Sjögren syndrome or other autoimmune diseases.[69] Furthermore, the heterogeneity of neurologic manifestations in primary Sjögren syndrome complicates the approach to treatment, which, ideally, should be directed toward the underlying neuropathologic mechanism. Treatment for peripheral sensory neuropathy will differ from that of mononeuritis multiplex and from that of the MS-like CNS involvement. The use of tricyclic antidepressant agents (such as amitriptyline and nortriptyline) for neuropathies is generally avoided because their anticholinergic side effects can contribute to existing sicca symptoms and may preclude achievement of a therapeutic effect. Symptomatic therapy for neuropathies often begins with gabapentin. The use of intravenous immunoglobulin may be beneficial for patients with peripheral motor and/or sensory neuropathies and peripheral demyelinating disorders that do not respond to glucocorticoids or to other immunosuppressive therapy.[70,71] Treatment options for autonomic neuropathy include fludrocortisone acetate or midodrine. Treatment of CNS involvement in primary Sjögren syndrome remains largely empirical, based on anecdotal reports and experience from treating the neurologic manifestations of SLE. Intravenous immunoglobulin, glucocorticoids, cyclophosphamide, rituximab, azathioprine, and methotrexate have all been used to treat CNS manifestations with limited success. Again, the approach to treatment in CNS manifestations of primary Sjögren syndrome depends on the underlying pathology, which may be vasculopathy, vasculitis, or demyelination.

REFERENCES

1. Garcia-Carrasco M, Ramos-Casals M, Rosas J, et al. Primary Sjogren syndrome: clinical and immunologic disease patterns in a cohort of 400 patients. Medicine (Baltimore) 2002;81(4):270–80.
2. Delalande S, de Seze J, Fauchais AL, et al. Neurologic manifestations in primary Sjogren syndrome: a study of 82 patients. Medicine (Baltimore) 2004;83(5): 280–91.
3. Mori K, Iijima M, Koike H, et al. The wide spectrum of clinical manifestations in Sjogren's syndrome-associated neuropathy. Brain 2005;128(Pt 11):2518–34.
4. Massara A, Bonazza S, Castellino G, et al. Central nervous system involvement in Sjogren's syndrome: unusual, but not unremarkable–clinical, serological characteristics and outcomes in a large cohort of Italian patients. Rheumatology (Oxford) 2010;49(8):1540–9.
5. Soliotis FC, Mavragani CP, Moutsopoulos HM. Central nervous system involvement in Sjogren's syndrome. Ann Rheum Dis 2004;63(6):616–20.
6. Moutsopoulos HM, Sarmas JH, Talal N. Is central nervous system involvement a systemic manifestation of primary Sjogren's syndrome? Rheum Dis Clin North Am 1993;19(4):909–12.
7. Vitali C, Bombardieri S, Moutsopoulos HM, et al. Assessment of the European classification criteria for Sjogren's syndrome in a series of clinically defined cases: results of a prospective multicentre study. The European Study Group on Diagnostic Criteria for Sjogren's syndrome. Ann Rheum Dis 1996;55(2): 116–21.
8. Fox RI, Robinson CA, Curd JG, et al. Sjogren's syndrome. Proposed criteria for classification. Arthritis Rheum 1986;29(5):577–85.
9. Vitali C, Bombardieri S, Jonsson R, et al. Classification criteria for Sjogren's syndrome: a revised version of the European criteria proposed by the American-European Consensus Group. Ann Rheum Dis 2002;61(6):554–8.
10. Barendregt PJ, van den Bent MJ, van Raaij-van den Aarssen VJ, et al. Involvement of the peripheral nervous system in primary Sjogren's syndrome. Ann Rheum Dis 2001;60(9):876–81.
11. Ioannidis JP, Moutsopoulos HM. Sjogren's syndrome: too many associations, too limited evidence. The enigmatic example of CNS involvement. Semin Arthritis Rheum 1999;29(1):1–3.
12. Miro J, Pena-Sagredo JL, Berciano J, et al. Prevalence of primary Sjogren's syndrome in patients with multiple sclerosis. Ann Neurol 1990;27(5):582–4.
13. Alexander EL, Provost TT, Stevens MB, et al. Neurologic complications of primary Sjogren's syndrome. Medicine (Baltimore) 1982;61(4):247–57.
14. Shen CC, Yang AC, Kuo BI, et al. Risk of psychiatric disorders following primary Sjogren syndrome: a nationwide population-based retrospective cohort study. J Rheumatol 2015;42(7):1203–8.
15. Harboe E, Tjensvoll AB, Maroni S, et al. Neuropsychiatric syndromes in patients with systemic lupus erythematosus and primary Sjogren syndrome: a comparative population-based study. Ann Rheum Dis 2009;68(10):1541–6.
16. Segal BM, Pogatchnik B, Holker E, et al. Primary Sjogren's syndrome: cognitive symptoms, mood, and cognitive performance. Acta Neurol Scand 2012;125(4): 272–8.
17. Westhoff G, Dorner T, Zink A. Fatigue and depression predict physician visits and work disability in women with primary Sjogren's syndrome: results from a cohort study. Rheumatology (Oxford) 2012;51(2):262–9.

18. Mellgren SI, Goransson LG, Omdal R. Primary Sjogren's syndrome associated neuropathy. Can J Neurol Sci 2007;34(3):280–7.
19. Griffin JW, Cornblath DR, Alexander E, et al. Ataxic sensory neuropathy and dorsal root ganglionitis associated with Sjogren's syndrome. Ann Neurol 1990;27(3): 304–15.
20. Mellgren SI, Conn DL, Stevens JC, et al. Peripheral neuropathy in primary Sjogren's syndrome. Neurology 1989;39(3):390–4.
21. Chai J, Herrmann DN, Stanton M, et al. Painful small-fiber neuropathy in Sjogren syndrome. Neurology 2005;65(6):925–7.
22. Font J, Ramos-Casals M, de la Red G, et al. Pure sensory neuropathy in primary Sjogren's syndrome. Longterm prospective followup and review of the literature. J Rheumatol 2003;30(7):1552–7.
23. Kawagashira Y, Koike H, Fujioka Y, et al. Differential, size-dependent sensory neuron involvement in the painful and ataxic forms of primary Sjogren's syndrome-associated neuropathy. J Neurol Sci 2012;319(1–2):139–46.
24. Birnbaum J, Duncan T, Owoyemi K, et al. Use of a novel high-resolution magnetic resonance neurography protocol to detect abnormal dorsal root Ganglia in Sjogren patients with neuropathic pain: case series of 10 patients and review of the literature. Medicine (Baltimore) 2014;93(3):121–34.
25. Pavlakis PP, Alexopoulos H, Kosmidis ML, et al. Peripheral neuropathies in Sjogren's syndrome: a critical update on clinical features and pathogenetic mechanisms. J Autoimmun 2012;39(1–2):27–33.
26. Sene D, Jallouli M, Lefaucheur JP, et al. Peripheral neuropathies associated with primary Sjogren syndrome: immunologic profiles of nonataxic sensory neuropathy and sensorimotor neuropathy. Medicine (Baltimore) 2011;90(2):133–8.
27. Birnbaum J. Peripheral nervous system manifestations of Sjogren syndrome: clinical patterns, diagnostic paradigms, etiopathogenesis, and therapeutic strategies. Neurologist 2010;16(5):287–97.
28. Brito-Zeron P, Akasbi M, Bosch X, et al. Classification and characterisation of peripheral neuropathies in 102 patients with primary Sjogren's syndrome. Clin Exp Rheumatol 2013;31(1):103–10.
29. Birnbaum J. Facial weakness, otalgia, and hemifacial spasm: a novel neurological syndrome in a case-series of 3 patients with rheumatic disease. Medicine (Baltimore) 2015;94(40):e1445.
30. Nascimento IS, Bonfa E, de Carvalho JF, et al. Clues for previously undiagnosed connective tissue disease in patients with trigeminal neuralgia. J Clin Rheumatol 2010;16(5):205–8.
31. Kumon Y, Kakigi A, Sugiura T. Clinical images: otalgia, an unusual complication of Sjogren's syndrome. Arthritis Rheum 2009;60(8):2542.
32. Freeman SR, Sheehan PZ, Thorpe MA, et al. Ear, nose, and throat manifestations of Sjogren's syndrome: retrospective review of a multidisciplinary clinic. J Otolaryngol 2005;34(1):20–4.
33. Mandl T, Bornmyr SV, Castenfors J, et al. Sympathetic dysfunction in patients with primary Sjogren's syndrome. J Rheumatol 2001;28(2):296–301.
34. Hammar O, Ohlsson B, Wollmer P, et al. Impaired gastric emptying in primary Sjogren's syndrome. J Rheumatol 2010;37(11):2313–8.
35. Sakakibara R, Hirano S, Asahina M, et al. Primary Sjogren's syndrome presenting with generalized autonomic failure. Eur J Neurol 2004;11(9):635–8.
36. Mandl T, Wollmer P, Manthorpe R, et al. Autonomic and orthostatic dysfunction in primary Sjogren's syndrome. J Rheumatol 2007;34(9):1869–74.

37. Cojocaru IM, Socoliuc G, Sapira V, et al. Primary Sjogren's syndrome or multiple sclerosis? Our experience concerning the dilemma of clinically isolated syndrome. Rom J Intern Med 2011;49(4):301–18.
38. Govoni M, Padovan M, Rizzo N, et al. CNS involvement in primary Sjogren's syndrome: prevalence, clinical aspects, diagnostic assessment and therapeutic approach. CNS Drugs 2001;15(8):597–607.
39. Rossi R, Valeria Saddi M. Subacute aseptic meningitis as neurological manifestation of primary Sjogren's syndrome. Clin Neurol Neurosurg 2006;108(7):688–91.
40. Lim JH, Chia FL, Lim TC, et al. A 62-year-old man with progressive weakness, multiple neurologic deficits, and hypernatremia. Arthritis Care Res (Hoboken) 2014;66(1):164–70.
41. Chen YW, Lee KC, Chang IW, et al. Sjogren's syndrome with acute cerebellar ataxia and massive lymphadenopathy: a case report. Acta Neurol Taiwan 2013; 22(2):81–6.
42. Wong S, Pollock AN, Burnham JM, et al. Acute cerebellar ataxia due to Sjogren syndrome. Neurology 2004;62(12):2332–3.
43. Delorme C, Cohen F, Hubsch C, et al. Chorea as the initial manifestation of Sjogren syndrome. Pediatr Neurol 2015;52(6):647–8.
44. Venegas Fanchke P, Sinning M, Miranda M. Primary Sjogren's syndrome presenting as a generalized chorea. Parkinsonism Relat Disord 2005;11(3):193–4.
45. Sawada J, Orimoto R, Misu T, et al. A case of pathology-proven neuromyelitis optica spectrum disorder with Sjogren syndrome manifesting aphasia and apraxia due to a localized cerebral white matter lesion. Mult Scler 2014;20(10):1413–6.
46. Lauvsnes MB, Maroni SS, Appenzeller S, et al. Memory dysfunction in primary Sjogren's syndrome is associated with anti-NR2 antibodies. Arthritis Rheum 2013;65(12):3209–17.
47. Yoshikawa K, Hatate J, Toratani N, et al. Prevalence of Sjogren's syndrome with dementia in a memory clinic. J Neurol Sci 2012;322(1–2):217–21.
48. Alexander EL. Neurologic disease in Sjogren's syndrome: mononuclear inflammatory vasculopathy affecting central/peripheral nervous system and muscle. A clinical review and update of immunopathogenesis. Rheum Dis Clin North Am 1993;19(4):869–908.
49. Alexander EL. Immunopathologic mechanisms of inflammatory vascular disease in primary Sjogren's syndrome–a model. Scand J Rheumatol Suppl 1986;61: 280–5.
50. Alexander EL, Lijewski JE, Jerdan MS, et al. Evidence of an immunopathogenic basis for central nervous system disease in primary Sjogren's syndrome. Arthritis Rheum 1986;29(10):1223–31.
51. Sanders ME, Alexander EL, Koski CL, et al. Detection of activated terminal complement (C5b-9) in cerebrospinal fluid from patients with central nervous system involvement of primary Sjogren's syndrome or systemic lupus erythematosus. J Immunol 1987;138(7):2095–9.
52. Molina R, Provost TT, Alexander EL. Peripheral inflammatory vascular disease in Sjogren's syndrome. Association with nervous system complications. Arthritis Rheum 1985;28(12):1341–7.
53. Alexander EL, Ranzenbach MR, Kumar AJ, et al. Anti-Ro(SS-A) autoantibodies in central nervous system disease associated with Sjogren's syndrome (CNS-SS): clinical, neuroimaging, and angiographic correlates. Neurology 1994;44(5): 899–908.

54. Manthorpe R, Manthorpe T, Sjoberg S. Magnetic resonance imaging of the brain in patients with primary Sjogren's syndrome. Scand J Rheumatol 1992;21(3): 148–9.
55. Segal BM, Mueller BA, Zhu X, et al. Disruption of brain white matter microstructure in primary Sjogren's syndrome: evidence from diffusion tensor imaging. Rheumatology (Oxford) 2010;49(8):1530–9.
56. Coates T, Slavotinek JP, Rischmueller M, et al. Cerebral white matter lesions in primary Sjogren's syndrome: a controlled study. J Rheumatol 1999;26(6):1301–5.
57. Pal B, Gibson C, Passmore J, et al. A study of headaches and migraine in Sjogren's syndrome and other rheumatic disorders. Ann Rheum Dis 1989;48(4): 312–6.
58. Tjensvoll AB, Harboe E, Goransson LG, et al. Headache in primary Sjogren's syndrome: a population-based retrospective cohort study. Eur J Neurol 2013;20(3): 558–63.
59. Druss BG, Walker ER. Mental disorders and medical comorbidity. Synth Proj Res Synth Rep 2011;(21):1–26.
60. Priori R, Minniti A, Antonazzo B, et al. Sleep quality in patients with primary Sjogren's syndrome. Clin Exp Rheumatol 2016;34(3):373–9.
61. Wong JK, Nortley R, Andrews T, et al. Psychiatric manifestations of primary Sjogren's syndrome: a case report and literature review. BMJ Case Rep 2014;2014 [pii:bcr2012008038].
62. Chiang CH, Liu CJ, Chen PJ, et al. Primary Sjogren's syndrome and risk of ischemic stroke: a nationwide study. Clin Rheumatol 2014;33(7):931–7.
63. Pasoto SG, Chakkour HP, Natalino RR, et al. Lupus anticoagulant: a marker for stroke and venous thrombosis in primary Sjogren's syndrome. Clin Rheumatol 2012;31(9):1331–8.
64. Lindvall B, Bengtsson A, Ernerudh J, et al. Subclinical myositis is common in primary Sjogren's syndrome and is not related to muscle pain. J Rheumatol 2002; 29(4):717–25.
65. Agarwal A, Sharma SK, Sinha S, et al. Primary Sjogren's syndrome presenting as flaccid quadriparesis. J Assoc Physicians India 2015;63(4):60–3.
66. Dasari S, Naha K, Vivek G, et al. Primary presentation with acute flaccid quadriparesis in Sjogren's syndrome sans sicca. BMJ Case Rep 2013;2013 [pii: bcr2012008172].
67. Cassese T, Kaplan E, Douglas V, et al. Getting to the right question. J Gen Intern Med 2013;28(9):1242–6.
68. de Seze J, Delalande S, Fauchais AL, et al. Myelopathies secondary to Sjögren's syndrome: treatment with monthly intravenous cyclophosphamide associated with corticosteroids. J Rheumatol 2006;33(4):709–11.
69. Ramos-Casals M, Garcia-Hernandez FJ, de Ramon E, et al. Off-label use of rituximab in 196 patients with severe, refractory systemic autoimmune diseases. Clin Exp Rheumatol 2010;28(4):468–76.
70. Takahashi Y, Takata T, Hoshino M, et al. Benefit of IVIG for long-standing ataxic sensory neuronopathy with Sjögren's syndrome. IV immunoglobulin. Neurology 2003;60(3):503–5.
71. Levy Y, Uziel Y, Zandman GG, et al. Intravenous immunoglobulins in peripheral neuropathy associated with vasculitis. Ann Rheum Dis 2003;62(12):1221–3.

Central Nervous System Manifestations of Systemic Lupus Erythematosus

Kashif Jafri, MD, Sarah L. Patterson, MD, Cristina Lanata, MD*

KEYWORDS

- Neuropsychiatric lupus • Anti-neuronal antibody • Blood–brain barrier dysfunction

KEY POINTS

- Neuropsychiatric systemic lupus erythematosus (NPSLE) is a severe manifestation of systemic lupus erythematosus (SLE) and can occur in about 40% of patients.
- Manifestations can be classified into diffuse manifestations (likely immune mediated) or focal manifestations (likely owing to vascular ischemia).
- Correct attribution of a neuropsychiatric event to active SLE is key and a challenging diagnostic dilemma.
- Important pathophysiologic aspects include the disruption of the blood–brain barrier, allowing passage of reactive antineuronal antibodies into the brain parenchyma.
- Sensitive biomarkers and imaging studies as well as high-quality evidence from clinical trials are needed to improve the diagnosis and management of NPSLE.

INTRODUCTION

Systemic lupus erythematosus (SLE) is a chronic systemic autoimmune disease characterized by autoantibody production and immune complex formation. It is the prototypic autoimmune disease, notable for its marked heterogeneity of disease manifestations. Internal organ involvement (such as the kidney and central nervous system) is characteristic of severe disease, and is what drives most of the disease morbidity and mortality.[1,2] Multiple mechanisms have been implicated in playing a role in the pathogenesis of neuropsychiatric SLE (NPSLE), including various arms of the immune system as well as nonimmune and environmental factors that could cause blood–brain barrier (BBB) dysfunction.[3] One of the most difficult aspects of central nervous system manifestations in clinical practice is their correct attribution to active

The authors have no financial disclosures and no conflicts of interest.
Division of Rheumatology, Department of Medicine, University of California, San Francisco, San Francisco, CA, USA
* Corresponding author. University of California, San Francisco, Box 0500, San Francisco, CA 94143.
E-mail address: Cristina.Lanata@ucsf.edu

SLE and this likely explains the wide range of reported prevalence of NPSLE (6.4%-93%).[4-6] Recent advances within the field include implementation of attribution models, which have been able to better define prevalence of NPSLE to 6% to 12% in the first year of diagnosis and a new calibrated overall prevalence of 19% to 38%.[7] In this review, we focus on central manifestations of NPSLE and summarize the latest understanding of disease pathogenesis, as well as specific clinical scenarios, treatment strategies, and outcomes.

DEFINITION AND CLASSIFICATION

In 1999, the American College of Rheumatology described 19 distinct phenomena, divided into central and peripheral manifestations, that are observed in NPSLE (**Box 1**). This schema was intended to establish a framework for research as well as clinical reporting[8]; however, it is nonspecific and not meant to be used as a diagnostic tool. Manifestations of NPSLE can be also classified into diffuse manifestations (such as psychosis and cognitive dysfunction) or focal manifestations (such as seizures and ischemic events), reflective of different disease mechanisms.

Box 1
Neuropsychiatric syndromes observed in systemic lupus erythematosus

Central nervous system

Aseptic meningitis

Cerebrovascular disease

Demyelinating syndrome

Headache (including migraine and benign intracranial hypertension)

Movement disorder (chorea)

Myelopathy

Seizure disorders

Acute confusional state

Anxiety disorder

Cognitive dysfunction

Mood disorder

Psychosis

Peripheral nervous system

Acute inflammatory demyelinating polyradiculoneuropathy (Guillain-Barre syndrome)

Autonomic disorder

Mononeuropathy, single or multiplex

Myasthenia gravis

Neuropathy, cranial

Plexopathy

Polyneuropathy

From The American College of Rheumatology nomenclature and case definitions for neuropsychiatric lupus syndromes. Arthritis Rheum 1999;42(4):599–608.

PATHOGENESIS OF NEUROPSYCHIATRIC SYSTEMIC LUPUS ERYTHEMATOSUS

The main histopathologic finding of NPSLE is a bland, noninflammatory microangiopathy in association with brain microinfarction. Microscopic findings in fatal NPSLE also include glial hyperplasia and diffuse neuronal and axonal loss.[9] True vasculitis, however, is rare. The innate and adaptive immune system has been implicated in the initiation of NPSLE, leading to the final pathway of microangiopathy and neuronal loss described.

Autoantibodies and Blood–Brain Barrier Dysfunction

SLE is known to produce a wide array of autoantibodies, with a total of 180 different autoantibodies described in sera of patients with SLE,[10] the majority of which are not tested routinely in clinical practice. The brain is thought to be protected from the circulating autoantibodies by the BBB; however, antibodies can access the brain parenchyma if the integrity of the barrier is disrupted. Therefore, a model of injury in NSPLE involves a 3-step process. First, antineuronal antibodies are produced in the periphery. Second, a breach in the BBB occurs, which may or may not be directly related to SLE, followed by antibody-mediated neuronal damage.

Sepsis, bacterial infections, trauma, brain ischemia, and stress have been shown to modulate and disrupt the integrity of the BBB. Specific agonists of endothelial receptors such as nicotine, caffeine, and cocaine have also been implicated.[11] A novel concept is that BBB disruption occurs in a regional fashion, according to the insult. For example, studies in rodents have shown that after bacterial lipopolysaccharide stimulation, there is an influx of IgG only in the hippocampus, and that systemic epinephrine administration will allow passage of IgG to the amygdala.[12,13] These findings offer a hypothesis for the varied manifestations observed in NPSLE because the effect of a potential antineuronal antibody depends on the location of the breach of the BBB, which in turn depends on the eliciting insult. There have been multiple antibodies associated with NPSLE. For the scope of this review, we will focus on anti-DNA and anti -N-methyl D Aspartate receptor antibodies, antiphospholipid antibodies, and anti-bosomal P antibodies.

Anti-DNA and Anti–N-Methyl-D-Aspartate Receptor Antibodies

Anti–double-stranded DNA (dsDNA) antibodies are the most common SLE-specific antibodies. A subset of anti-dsDNA antibodies have been shown to cross-react with the NMDA and are called anti-DNA/NMDA antibodies.[14] Elegant studies have shown that both murine and human anti-DNA/NMDA antibodies bind preferably to the active NMDA receptor, causing excess calcium influx, overstimulation, neuronal dysfunction and cell death.[15] This specific anti-DNA/NMDA antibody is found in 30% to 40% of patients with SLE with anti-dsDNA antibodies. The effects of this antibody can be long lasting; rodent studies have shown that neurons continue to undergo a loss of dendritic processes, or increased neuronal pruning, after antibody is no longer detected in brain tissue. These alterations have been shown to correlate with impairment of spatial memory in mice.[16] In patients with NPSLE, the presence of anti-DNA/NMDA antibodies in the CSF, but not in serum, correlate with active diffuse NSPLE manifestations, such as psychosis or acute confusional state.[17] This corroborates the importance of BBB disruption in the development of NPSLE.

Anti-P Antibodies

Anti–ribosomal-P antibodies have been associated with variable consistency in diffuse manifestations of NPSLE such as psychosis.[18] They were initially identified as binding to the C-terminal regions of 3 ribosomal P proteins.[11] However, these antibodies also cross-react with a plasma membrane protein of unknown function called neuronal surface P antigen, which is expressed exclusively in neurons.[19] Studies have shown that passive transfer of human anti-P antibodies induced depression-like behavior and memory impairment in mice. In vitro and in vivo studies have revealed that anti-P antibodies induce neuronal death through an excitatory glutamic pathway mediated by neuronal surface P antigen, involving the NMDA receptor.

Antiphospholipid Antibodies

Antiphospholipid antibodies have been associated primarily with focal manifestations of NPSLE, such as stroke, seizures, and transverse myelitis (TM). They are thought to contribute to pathogenesis owing to their prothrombotic properties, resulting in vasculopathy and microangiopathy and leading to ischemia and neuronal cell death. However, they have also been associated with cognitive dysfunction.[18] Observational studies show a high prevalence of aPL positivity (up to 73%) among patients with SLE-associated TM.[20,21] The anterior medial longitudinal arterial trunk is smaller in the thoracic region as compared with the cervical and lumbar regions. The midthoracic spinal cord, therefore, represents a "watershed area" that is more vulnerable to arterial insufficiency in the setting of thrombotic disease. The observed association between aPL antibodies and TM in patients with SLE, as well as the predilection for thoracic cord involvement, have led to the hypothesis that aPL-induced arterial occlusion contributes to the pathogenesis of this syndrome.[22]

Cytokines

Inflammatory mediators such as tumor necrosis factor, IL-6, IL-1, interferon-γ, and tumor necrosis factor–related weak inducer of apoptosis have been shown to cause BBB dysfunction.[3] There is also evidence of intrathecal production of cytokines such as IL-6, IL-2, IL-10, and plasminogen activator inhibitor 1 in patients with NPSLE compared with patients with SLE who did not exhibit overt neuropsychiatric involvement.[23–26] The source of intrathecal cytokine production is thought to be from activated microglia in response to antineuronal antibodies.[27,28]

CLINICAL MANIFESTATIONS
Diffuse Manifestations

Headaches and mood disorders are the most frequent neuropsychiatric complaints among patients with SLE, but are uncommonly directly attributed to SLE. Recent evidence does not support an increased rate of headaches among patients with SLE compared with non-SLE individuals, and headache has not been associated with disease activity, use of steroids or immunosuppressants, or specific autoantibodies. Furthermore, the majority of headaches resolved over time, independent of lupus-specific therapies.[29] In a recent study in an international SLE inception cohort, mood disorders were described in 232 patients (12.7%), of which 98 (38.2%) were attributed to SLE, with an estimated cumulative incidence of any mood disorder after 10 years of 17.7%.[30] The primary conclusion of this study was that most mood disorders were not attributed to SLE.

Cognitive Dysfunction

Cognitive dysfunction, so-called brain fog, is commonly reported by patients with SLE. Cognitive disorders are a category of mental health disorders that primarily affect learning, memory, perception, and problem solving. They are reported at a higher frequency in patients with SLE in comparison with healthy controls[31]; however, they are not specific to SLE, and are also frequently observed in depression[32] and in many chronic illnesses. Cognitive dysfunction should be confirmed by formal neuropsychological assessment. There are several tools that are used to screen for cognitive dysfunction; however, a commonly cited tool is the Automated Neuropsychological Assessment Metrics,[31] which has been shown to be a sensitive test for the detection of cognitive dysfunction in patients with SLE. Although cognitive dysfunction has been associated with anti-DNA/NMDA antibodies as well as aPL antibodies, evidence supporting the use of anticoagulation, NMDA receptor antagonists, or other immunosuppressants for the treatment of cognitive dysfunction is lacking.[18,33] Treatment of other factors that are known to affect cognition such as depression, sleep deprivation, and medications should be appropriately assessed and managed.

Acute Confusional State and Psychosis

Acute confusional state and psychosis are diffuse neuropsychiatric manifestations that often occur without any associated structural pathology.[34] They are considered relatively uncommon manifestations (about 1%–5%), although the prevalence of psychosis has been found to be as high as approximately 11% in some studies.[6,35,36] Acute confusional state is characterized by an acute disturbance in consciousness ranging from delirium to coma. Psychosis is characterized by delusions (false beliefs) and/or hallucinations (perceptions in the absence of external stimuli); most episodes of lupus psychosis resolve within 2 to 4 weeks.[6,34] Schizophrenia, substance abuse, adverse effects from glucocorticoids, and metabolic or endocrine disturbances should be evaluated for in a patient with SLE presenting with psychosis. Importantly, steroid-induced psychiatric disease typically presents as a mood disorder rather than as true psychosis.[6,37] Glucocorticoids and other immunosuppressive therapy may be considered in severe cases of acute confusional state or SLE-associated psychosis, especially in the presence of generalized SLE disease activity.[6] Antipsychotic treatment may be used in SLE-associated psychosis as clinically indicated, but should only be used in refractory cases of acute confusional state when other interventions have been ineffective.[6]

Posterior Reversible Encephalopathy Syndrome

Posterior reversible encephalopathy syndrome (PRES) is characterized by headaches, altered mental status, visual disturbances, and seizures with radiographic lesions in the posterior cerebral white matter.[38,39] Patients with SLE are at increased risk for PRES, but it is not considered a true manifestation of NPSLE. Rather, its clinical presentation can mimic manifestations of NPSLE such as seizure. The pathophysiology of PRES is not well-understood, but one hypothesized mechanism focuses on cerebral autoregulatory failure and hyperperfusion in the setting of hypertension, with a possible contribution from additional endothelial injury from other risk factors. Dysregulation of arteriolar constriction is suspected to lead to relative cerebral arteriolar vasodilation, which results in extravasation of fluid and protein into the brain parenchyma.[38,40,41] Because the sympathetic innervation is relatively poor in the vertebrobasilar system, the posterior circulation is more susceptible to this vasogenic edema.[38,40,41]

Risk factors for PRES include hypertension, uremia, preeclampsia, eclampsia, SLE, human immunodeficiency virus infection, thrombotic thrombocytopenic purpura, solid organ transplantation, and the use of certain drugs (eg, corticosteroids, tacrolimus, cyclosporine, interferon-alfa, intravenous immunoglobulin, and cyclophosphamide).[38,39] PRES is an uncommon complication in SLE, but patients with SLE may be at an increased risk for PRES for multiple reasons, including endothelial dysfunction in SLE, the use of cytotoxic drugs, and the increased prevalence of comorbidities such as hypertension and renal disease.[42,43] MRI studies help to confirm the diagnosis of PRES with characteristic findings of diffuse hyperintense signals predominantly in the posterior parietal and occipital lobes on T2- and fluid-attenuated inversion recovery—weighted images.[40,41] Early diagnosis of PRES is critical, because most patients experience complete clinical and radiographic resolution with prompt antihypertensive treatment and withdrawal of the suspected inciting immunosuppressive drug.[39] The relationship between SLE and PRES is an important area for future study because the mechanism and risk of PRES in SLE are poorly understood. It is not clear whether PRES may be a manifestation of active SLE that could ultimately require intensification of immunosuppressive therapy in a certain subset of patients.[42,44–46]

FOCAL MANIFESTATIONS
Stroke

It is estimated that 3% to 15% of patients with SLE will have a stroke at some point during their disease course.[47–50] The risk of stroke among lupus patients is increased relative to the general population, although the amount of risk conferred remains controversial. Whereas observational data from cohort studies suggests a relative risk as high as 8,[51] a large study using United States hospital registry data reported a relative risk of 1.5.[52] When evaluating the risk of stroke subtypes, patients with lupus are at an increased risk of ischemic stroke and cerebral hemorrhage, but not subarachnoid hemorrhage, compared with the general population.[52]

Stroke in patients with lupus results from a variety of pathophysiologic mechanisms including thromboembolic disease, accelerated atherosclerosis, vascular inflammation, and hypercoagulable states.[53–56] In addition to traditional Framingham risk factors, variables associated with increased risk of stroke include the presence of aPLs, high disease activity, and valvular disease such as Libman-Sacks endocarditis.[56–58] The management is similar to that of non–SLE-related strokes, including aggressive cardiovascular risk reduction and anticoagulation in cases deemed secondary to hypercoagulable conditions such as antiphospholipid syndrome.[54] Immunosuppression is not recommended unless indicated based on clinical and laboratory assessments consistent with high disease activity.

Seizure

Seizures affect an estimated 8% to 18% of patient with lupus.[59] They can occur at any time, but most commonly occur early in the disease course, with roughly one-half of affected patients experiencing their first seizure within the first year after diagnosis.[60,61] Generalized, complex partial, and simple partial seizures attributed to lupus have all been described.[61–65] In a cohort of 600 multiethnic patients with SLE, seizures contributed to accrual of disease damage, but not to an increased risk of mortality.[66] A number of studies have evaluated risk and protective factors for development of seizures in the setting of SLE. Variables associated with increased risk include younger age, higher disease activity, Hispanic and African American ethnicity, previous stroke, and a previous episode of psychosis.[66,67] Additionally, there seems to be an increased risk in patients with anti-Smith antibodies,[68] as well as in those with antiphospholipid antibodies.[64,69] In contrast, the presence of the anti-La antibody and the use of antimalarial drugs have both been shown to have a protective role in seizure occurrence.[66,70] Treatment requires a multidisciplinary approach, including evaluation by a neurologist and institution of antiepileptic therapy in cases deemed at high risk for recurrence.

Transverse Myelitis

TM is a rare manifestation of SLE, with an estimated prevalence in patients with SLE of 1% to 2%.[71] Diagnosis requires the presence of bilateral neurologic deficits referable to the spinal cord that develop over 4 hours to 21 days, as well as objective evidence of an active inflammatory process demonstrated by the presence of elevated protein and/or white blood cells on cerebrospinal fluid (CSF) analysis or gadolinium enhancement of the spinal cord on MRI.[72,73] In a metaanalysis of 105 cases of lupus myelitis, most patients developed TM either as the initial manifestation of SLE (46%) or within 5 years of the diagnosis, and the most common clinical presentation was a thoracic sensory level.[20] Other characteristic clinical manifestations include symmetric motor weakness and bladder dysfunction.

TM presents a challenging diagnostic and treatment dilemma, because there is a variety of underlying diseases known to cause the syndrome, and appropriate treatment is both time-sensitive and depends on the underlying etiology.[21,74] The diagnostic evaluation should include spine MRI with and without contrast, brain MRI, CSF analysis, and testing for serum aquaporin-4 autoantibody (AQP4-IgG). The most commonly reported spine MRI findings are long segment T2 hyperintensity, cord expansion or swelling, and gadolinium enhancement on T1-weighted sequences.[73] The presence of serum AQP4-IgG has a high specificity (85%–99%) for neuromyelitis optica spectrum disorder (NMOSD), which can occur concomitantly with SLE or in isolation.[75] Diagnosis and management of NMOSD is discussed in detail elsewhere in this issue.

The goal of treatment is to maximize the probability of neurologic recovery and minimize long-term disability. Given the rarity of lupus myelitis, there are no randomized controlled trials to guide treatment decisions. However, observational data suggest improved outcomes in patients treated with high-dose steroids, for example, methylprednisolone 1000 mg intravenously for 3 consecutive days followed by an oral steroid taper. Because inflammatory etiologies represent the majority of causes of TM, once infectious etiologies have been excluded, high- dose intravenous glucocorticoids should be initiated without delay.[76,77] Steroid-sparing immunosuppression is dictated in part by AQP4-IgG status and suspicion for concomitant NMOSD; cyclophosphamide is a first-line therapy for isolated lupus myelitis, whereas the efficacy data for rituximab is superior in patients with NMOSD.[78–80]

DIAGNOSTIC APPROACH AND DIFFERENTIAL DIAGNOSIS OF NEUROPSYCHIATRIC SYSTEMIC LUPUS ERYTHEMATOSUS

In general, the diagnostic workup of neuropsychiatric symptoms in patients with SLE should be similar to that of patients without SLE with the same symptoms.[81] A careful history regarding medications, comorbidities, and illicit drug use should be taken. It is very important to establish not only a diagnosis of SLE, but also to evaluate SLE disease activity apart from the presenting neuropsychiatric manifestation. This process aids in attributing the event to SLE or to non-SLE factors, although disease activity has correlated most directly with diffuse NPSLE. The initial laboratory assessment should include a complete blood count, comprehensive metabolic panel, thyroid studies, anti-dsDNA, erythrocyte sedimentation rate, C-reactive protein, C3, C4, and urinalysis. The specific diagnostic tests ordered depend on the potential focal or diffuse neuropsychiatric manifestations that are being considered. For example, aPL studies, including anticardiolipin antibodies, β2-glycoprotein 1 antibodies, and lupus anticoagulant assays, may provide useful diagnostic information in patients with focal manifestations such as stroke.[82]

It is crucial to exclude other etiologies, such as infections, medication adverse effects, and metabolic abnormalities before ascribing symptoms to NPSLE. Infections are especially important to exclude in immunosuppressed patients with SLE, and an infectious workup including blood cultures, urine culture, a chest radiograph, CSF culture, and CSF polymerase chain reaction for herpes simplex virus and JC virus should be considered if indicated clinically. In the absence of infection, CSF abnormalities, such as an elevated white blood cell count, protein, and IgG index or a decreased glucose level, may be suggestive of active NPSLE, but are not necessarily diagnostic. One way to assess for BBB integrity is calculating an albumin concentration gradient between CSF and plasma (Q_{alb}).[3] Albumin is not synthesized intrathecally; therefore, it can serve as an indicator of a relatively large leakage across the BBB. However, it lacks sensitivity for small and transient leakages.[83]

Electrophysiologic studies, neuropsychological assessment, and neuroimaging can be considered to evaluate whether a specific clinical manifestation is attributable to NPSLE.[18] Electroencephalography can be useful in diagnosing a seizure disorder; neuropsychological testing in assessing cognitive function; and MRI (T1/T2, fluid-attenuating inversion recovery, diffusion-weighted imaging, enhanced T1 sequence) in assessing brain structure and function.[6] The average sensitivity of MRI in active NPSLE is about 57%, and although the most common pathologic pattern is punctate hyperintense T2-weighted focal lesions in subcortical and periventricular white matter, these findings are often seen in patients without active NPSLE.[6] More advanced neuroimaging techniques using MRI and nuclear imaging (PET and single photon emission computed tomography) require further validation with respect to their clinical usefulness in NPSLE. (**Fig. 1**) showed MRI findings of select manifestations of CNS lupus.

Given the challenges in ascribing nonspecific neuropsychiatric symptoms to SLE, algorithms have been proposed to assist in accurate attribution.[84] One such attribution model was recently developed and validated by Bortoluzzi and colleagues[85] on behalf of the Study Group for NPSLE of the Italian Society of Rheumatology. It addressed 4 themes, including the temporal relationship of neuropsychiatric events to the diagnosis of SLE, identification of common or minor neuropsychiatric events, recognition of confounding factors (ie, alternative etiologies or non-SLE contributing factors derived from American College of Radiology case definitions), and recognition of favoring factors (ie, clinical and nonclinical variables derived from European League Against Rheumatism recommendations and an expert panel).[81] Although significant progress has been made in the development of attribution models, multidisciplinary clinical assessment remains critical in the accurate attribution of neuropsychiatric events to SLE or to other causes.[86]

TREATMENT STRATEGIES OF NEUROPSYCHIATRIC SYSTEMIC LUPUS ERYTHEMATOSUS

The evidence for treatment of NPSLE is limited given the heterogeneity of the disease, study variation in treatment doses and outcome measures, and the absence of high-quality randomized, controlled trials.[87] Treatment strategies differ depending on the specific presenting manifestation, the presumptive pathophysiologic mechanism, and a clinical assessment of its severity. Symptomatic treatment is a cornerstone of the therapeutic strategy for many NPSLE manifestations, such as antidepressants for depression, antiepileptic agents for seizures, and antipsychotic agents for psychosis. Antiplatelet therapy and anticoagulation should be considered in patients with SLE whose neuropsychiatric manifestation is attributable to thrombosis. The treatment of any underlying infections and relevant comorbidities that may contribute to neuropsychiatric symptoms, such as hypertension and diabetes mellitus, is also important.

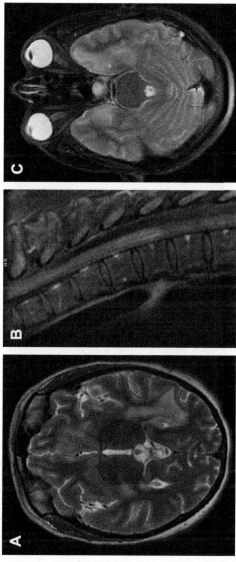

Fig. 1. MRI findings in central nervous system lupus. (A) Acute confusional state. Multiple T2 hyperintense periventricular white matter involvement in bilateral temporal and frontal lobes in a patient with central nervous system lupus presenting with an acute confusional state. (B) Lupus myelitis. Abnormal T2 prolongation is noted within the thoracic spinal cord extending from T3 through the T6 level. (C) Encephalopathy with severe cognitive impairment. T2 hyperintensity involving the medial aspect of the temporal lobes bilaterally.

For mild to moderate neuropsychiatric manifestations that are attributed to persistent autoimmune or inflammatory mechanisms, the use of glucocorticoids and immunosuppressants such as azathioprine or mycophenolate mofetil should be considered.[84] For any life-threatening or severe neuropsychiatric manifestation that is attributable to autoimmune or inflammatory mechanisms and may result in permanent neurologic deficits (eg, TM), high-dose corticosteroids and aggressive immunosuppressive therapy with cyclophosphamide should be initiated promptly. In a randomized, controlled trial of 32 patients with SLE with incident onset of severe neuropsychiatric manifestations at 2 tertiary care centers in Mexico City, a statistically significant treatment response (defined as a 20% improvement from basal condition by clinical, serologic, and specific neurologic measures) was found in 94.7% of patients using cyclophosphamide compared with 46.2% in the methylprednisolone group at 24 months (relative risk, 2.05; 95% CI, 1.13–3.73).[88,89] Cyclophosphamide has been demonstrated to prevent relapses of NPSLE and to have a steroid-sparing effect, but it is also important to note that it has been associated with cumulative damage, ovarian failure, and the development of cervical intraepithelial neoplasia.[87] Rituximab, intravenous immunoglobulin, and plasma exchange are potential therapeutic options that can be considered in refractory cases of NPSLE.[81,90,91] In the future, randomized, controlled trials with large numbers of well-characterized patients with SLE are necessary to develop a more systematic, evidence-based approach to the management of NPSLE.

OUTCOMES

There are few observational studies regarding long-term outcomes of NPSLE, and data come primarily from the Systemic Lupus Erythematosus International Collaborating Clinics (SLICC) cohort. After follow-up of up to 7 years (average, 3.5), 15% of neuropsychiatric events were resolved at each annual assessment; however, most persisted.[92] Higher global disease activity was associated with worse short-term outcomes (<5 months), but NPSLE events attributed to SLE had better outcome scores than events attributed to non-SLE causes.[93] Regardless of the cause or attribution, NPSLE manifestations in patients with SLE are associated with a substantial negative impact on health-related quality of life.[94]

SUMMARY

NPSLE remains a diagnostic and therapeutic challenge in patients with SLE. The correct attribution of neuropsychiatric manifestations to active SLE or to SLE-related factors is of paramount importance. Despite increasing understanding of the disease pathogenesis, clinicians still lack appropriate diagnostic biomarkers and sensitive imaging studies to fully aid in the diagnosis. Furthermore, it seems that the window for treatment might be much earlier than actual disease manifestations, based on recent animal studies. Current treatment strategies are largely empiric, and are guided by treatment approaches used in other SLE manifestations as well as other rheumatologic diseases. A further understanding of disease pathogenesis will hopefully aid in the design and implementation of clinical trials, which are mostly lacking.

REFERENCES

1. Zirkzee EJ, Huizinga TW, Bollen EL, et al. Mortality in neuropsychiatric systemic lupus erythematosus (NPSLE). Lupus 2014;23:31–8.

2. Cervera R, Khamashta MA, Font J, et al. Morbidity and mortality in systemic lupus erythematosus during a 5-year period. A multicenter prospective study of 1,000 patients. European Working Party on Systemic Lupus Erythematosus. Medicine (Baltimore) 1999;78:167–75.

3. Stock AD, Wen J, Putterman C. Neuropsychiatric lupus, the blood brain barrier, and the TWEAK/Fn14 Pathway. Front Immunol 2013;4:484.

4. Borowoy AM, Pope JE, Silverman E, et al. Neuropsychiatric lupus: the prevalence and autoantibody associations depend on the definition: results from the 1000 faces of lupus cohort. Semin Arthritis Rheum 2012;42:179–85.

5. Unterman A, Nolte JE, Boaz M, et al. Neuropsychiatric syndromes in systemic lupus erythematosus: a meta-analysis. Semin Arthritis Rheum 2011;41:1–11.

6. Bertsias GK, Ioannidis JP, Aringer M, et al. EULAR recommendations for the management of systemic lupus erythematosus with neuropsychiatric manifestations: report of a task force of the EULAR standing committee for clinical affairs. Ann Rheum Dis 2010;69:2074–82.

7. Hanly JG. Attribution in the assessment of nervous system disease in SLE. Rheumatology (Oxford) 2015;54:755–6.

8. The American College of Rheumatology nomenclature and case definitions for neuropsychiatric lupus syndromes. Arthritis Rheum 1999;42:599–608.

9. Sibbitt WL Jr, Brooks WM, Kornfeld M, et al. Magnetic resonance imaging and brain histopathology in neuropsychiatric systemic lupus erythematosus. Semin Arthritis Rheum 2010;40:32–52.

10. Yaniv G, Twig G, Shor DB-A, et al. A volcanic explosion of autoantibodies in systemic lupus erythematosus: a diversity of 180 different antibodies found in SLE patients. Autoimmun Rev 2015;14:75–9.

11. Brimberg L, Mader S, Fujieda Y, et al. Antibodies as mediators of brain pathology. Trends Immunol 2015;36:709–24.

12. Huerta PT, Kowal C, DeGiorgio LA, et al. Immunity and behavior: antibodies alter emotion. Proc Natl Acad Sci U S A 2006;103:678–83.

13. Kowal C, Degiorgio LA, Lee JY, et al. Human lupus autoantibodies against NMDA receptors mediate cognitive impairment. Proc Natl Acad Sci U S A 2006;103:19854–9.

14. DeGiorgio LA, Konstantinov KN, Lee SC, et al. A subset of lupus anti-DNA antibodies cross-reacts with the NR2 glutamate receptor in systemic lupus erythematosus. Nat Med 2001;7:1189–93.

15. Faust TW, Chang EH, Kowal C, et al. Neurotoxic lupus autoantibodies alter brain function through two distinct mechanisms. Proc Natl Acad Sci U S A 2010;107:18569–74.

16. Chang EH, Volpe BT, Mackay M, et al. Selective impairment of spatial cognition caused by autoantibodies to the N-Methyl-D-Aspartate receptor. EBioMedicine 2015;2:755–64.

17. Arinuma Y, Yanagida T, Hirohata S. Association of cerebrospinal fluid anti-NR2 glutamate receptor antibodies with diffuse neuropsychiatric systemic lupus erythematosus. Arthritis Rheum 2008;58:1130–5.

18. Hanly JG. Diagnosis and management of neuropsychiatric SLE. Nat Rev Rheumatol 2014;10:338–47.

19. Matus S, Burgos PV, Bravo-Zehnder M, et al. Antiribosomal-P autoantibodies from psychiatric lupus target a novel neuronal surface protein causing calcium influx and apoptosis. J Exp Med 2007;204:3221–34.

20. Kovacs B, Lafferty TL, Brent LH, et al. Transverse myelopathy in systemic lupus erythematosus: an analysis of 14 cases and review of the literature. Ann Rheum Dis 2000;59:120–4.

21. D'Cruz DP, Mellor-Pita S, Joven B, et al. Transverse myelitis as the first manifestation of systemic lupus erythematosus or lupus-like disease: good functional outcome and relevance of antiphospholipid antibodies. J Rheumatol 2004;31: 280–5.

22. Lavalle C, Pizarro S, Drenkard C, et al. Transverse myelitis: a manifestation of systemic lupus erythematosus strongly associated with antiphospholipid antibodies. J Rheumatol 1990;17:34–7.

23. Hirohata S, Miyamoto T. Elevated levels of interleukin-6 in cerebrospinal fluid from patients with systemic lupus erythematosus and central nervous system involvement. Arthritis Rheum 1990;33:644–9.

24. Hirohata S, Hayakawa K. Enhanced interleukin-6 messenger RNA expression by neuronal cells in a patient with neuropsychiatric systemic lupus erythematosus. Arthritis Rheum 1999;42:2729–30.

25. Shiozawa S, Kuroki Y, Kim M, et al. Interferon-alpha in lupus psychosis. Arthritis Rheum 1992;35:417–22.

26. Kwiecinski J, Klak M, Trysberg E, et al. Relationship between elevated cerebrospinal fluid levels of plasminogen activator inhibitor 1 and neuronal destruction in patients with neuropsychiatric systemic lupus erythematosus. Arthritis Rheum 2009;60:2094–101.

27. Sato S, Kawashima H, Hoshika A, et al. Clinical analysis of anti-NR2 glutamate receptor antibodies and interleukin-6 with neuropsychiatric systemic lupus erythematosus. Rheumatology (Oxford) 2011;50:2142–4.

28. Santer DM, Yoshio T, Minota S, et al. Potent induction of IFN-alpha and chemokines by autoantibodies in the cerebrospinal fluid of patients with neuropsychiatric lupus. J Immunol 2009;182:1192–201.

29. Hanly JG, Urowitz MB, O'Keeffe AG, et al. Headache in systemic lupus erythematosus: results from a prospective, international inception cohort study. Arthritis Rheum 2013;65:2887–97.

30. Hanly JG, Su L, Urowitz MB, et al. Mood Disorders in Systemic Lupus Erythematosus: results From an International Inception Cohort Study. Arthritis Rheum 2015; 67:1837–47.

31. Hanly JG, Su L, Omisade A, et al. Screening for cognitive impairment in systemic lupus erythematosus. J Rheumatol 2012;39:1371–7.

32. Clark M, DiBenedetti D, Perez V. Cognitive dysfunction and work productivity in major depressive disorder. Expert Rev Pharmacoecon Outcomes Res 2016;16: 455–63.

33. Petri M, Naqibuddin M, Sampedro M, et al. Memantine in systemic lupus erythematosus: a randomized, double-blind placebo-controlled trial. Semin Arthritis Rheum 2011;41:194–202.

34. Jeltsch-David H, Muller S. Neuropsychiatric systemic lupus erythematosus: pathogenesis and biomarkers. Nat Rev Neurol 2014;10:579–96.

35. Abdel-Nasser AM, Ghaleb RM, Mahmoud JA, et al. Association of anti-ribosomal P protein antibodies with neuropsychiatric and other manifestations of systemic lupus erythematosus. Clin Rheumatol 2008;27:1377–85.

36. Appenzeller S, Cendes F, Costallat LT. Acute psychosis in systemic lupus erythematosus. Rheumatol Int 2008;28:237–43.

37. Chau SY, Mok CC. Factors predictive of corticosteroid psychosis in patients with systemic lupus erythematosus. Neurology 2003;61:104–7.

38. Ferreira TS, Reis F, Appenzeller S. Posterior reversible encephalopathy syndrome and association with systemic lupus erythematosus. Lupus 2016;25:1369–76.
39. Magnano MD, Bush TM, Herrera I, et al. Reversible posterior leukoencephalopathy in patients with systemic lupus erythematosus. Semin Arthritis Rheum 2006;35:396–402.
40. Min L, Zwerling J, Ocava LC, et al. Reversible posterior leukoencephalopathy in connective tissue diseases. Semin Arthritis Rheum 2006;35:388–95.
41. Mak A, Chan BP, Yeh IB, et al. Neuropsychiatric lupus and reversible posterior leucoencephalopathy syndrome: a challenging clinical dilemma. Rheumatology (Oxford) 2008;47:256–62.
42. Lai CC, Chen WS, Chang YS, et al. Clinical features and outcomes of posterior reversible encephalopathy syndrome in patients with systemic lupus erythematosus. Arthritis Care Res (Hoboken) 2013;65:1766–74.
43. Merayo-Chalico J, Apodaca E, Barrera-Vargas A, et al. Clinical outcomes and risk factors for posterior reversible encephalopathy syndrome in systemic lupus erythematosus: a multicentric case-control study. J Neurol Neurosurg Psychiatr 2016;87:287–94.
44. Barber CE, Leclerc R, Gladman DD, et al. Posterior reversible encephalopathy syndrome: an emerging disease manifestation in systemic lupus erythematosus. Semin Arthritis Rheum 2011;41:353–63.
45. Shaharir SS, Remli R, Marwan AA, et al. Posterior reversible encephalopathy syndrome in systemic lupus erythematosus: pooled analysis of the literature reviews and report of six new cases. Lupus 2013;22:492–6.
46. Budhoo A, Mody GM. The spectrum of posterior reversible encephalopathy in systemic lupus erythematosus. Clin Rheumatol 2015;34:2127–34.
47. Futrell N, Millikan C. Frequency, etiology, and prevention of stroke in patients with systemic lupus erythematosus. Stroke 1989;20:583–91.
48. Kitagawa Y, Gotoh F, Koto A, et al. Stroke in systemic lupus erythematosus. Stroke 1990;21:1533–9.
49. Manzi S, Selzer F, Sutton-Tyrrell K, et al. Prevalence and risk factors of carotid plaque in women with systemic lupus erythematosus. Arthritis Rheum 1999;42: 51–60.
50. Sibley JT, Olszynski WP, Decoteau WE, et al. The incidence and prognosis of central nervous system disease in systemic lupus erythematosus. J Rheumatol 1992; 19:47–52.
51. Esdaile JM, Abrahamowicz M, Grodzicky T, et al. Traditional Framingham risk factors fail to fully account for accelerated atherosclerosis in systemic lupus erythematosus. Arthritis Rheum 2001;44:2331–7.
52. Krishnan E. Stroke subtypes among young patients with systemic lupus erythematosus. Am J Med 2005;118:1415.
53. Jennekens FG, Kater L. The central nervous system in systemic lupus erythematosus. Part 2. Pathogenetic mechanisms of clinical syndromes: a literature investigation. Rheumatology (Oxford) 2002;41:619–30.
54. Timlin H, Petri M. Transient ischemic attack and stroke in systemic lupus erythematosus. Lupus 2013;22:1251–8.
55. Mitsias P, Levine SR. Large cerebral vessel occlusive disease in systemic lupus erythematosus. Neurology 1994;44:385–93.
56. Roldan CA, Gelgand EA, Qualls CR, et al. Valvular heart disease as a cause of cerebrovascular disease in patients with systemic lupus erythematosus. Am J Cardiol 2005;95:1441–7.

57. Mikdashi J, Handwerger B, Langenberg P, et al. Baseline disease activity, hyperlipidemia, and hypertension are predictive factors for ischemic stroke and stroke severity in systemic lupus erythematosus. Stroke 2007;38:281–5.
58. Greenberg BM. The neurologic manifestations of systemic lupus erythematosus. Neurologist 2009;15:115–21.
59. Muscal E, Brey RL. Neurologic manifestations of systemic lupus erythematosus in children and adults. Neurol Clin 2010;28:61–73.
60. Hanly JG, Urowitz MB, Su L, et al. Seizure disorders in systemic lupus erythematosus results from an international, prospective, inception cohort study. Ann Rheum Dis 2012;71:1502–9.
61. Gonzalez-Duarte A, Cantu-Brito CG, Ruano-Calderon L, et al. Clinical description of seizures in patients with systemic lupus erythematosus. Eur Neurol 2008;59:320–3.
62. Joseph FG, Lammie GA, Scolding NJ. CNS lupus: a study of 41 patients. Neurology 2007;69:644–54.
63. Glanz BI, Schur PH, Khoshbin S. EEG abnormalities in systemic lupus erythematosus. Clin Electroencephalogr 1998;29:128–31.
64. Appenzeller S, Cendes F, Costallat LT. Epileptic seizures in systemic lupus erythematosus. Neurology 2004;63:1808–12.
65. Mayes B, Brey RL. Evaluation and treatment of seizures in patients with systemic lupus erythematosus. J Clin Rheumatol 1996;2:336–45.
66. Andrade RM, Alarcon GS, Gonzalez LA, et al. Seizures in patients with systemic lupus erythematosus: data from LUMINA, a multiethnic cohort (LUMINA LIV). Ann Rheum Dis 2008;67:829–34.
67. Ramsey-Goldman R, Alarcon GS, McGwin G, et al. Time to seizure occurrence and damage in PROFILE, a multi-ethnic systemic lupus erythematosus cohort. Lupus 2008;17:177–84.
68. Mikdashi J, Krumholz A, Handwerger B. Factors at diagnosis predict subsequent occurrence of seizures in systemic lupus erythematosus. Neurology 2005;64:2102–7.
69. Herranz MT, Rivier G, Khamashta MA, et al. Association between antiphospholipid antibodies and epilepsy in patients with systemic lupus erythematosus. Arthritis Rheum 1994;37:568–71.
70. Malik S, Bruner GR, Williams-Weese C, et al. Presence of anti-La autoantibody is associated with a lower risk of nephritis and seizures in lupus patients. Lupus 2007;16:863–6.
71. Theodoridou A, Settas L. Demyelination in rheumatic diseases. Postgrad Med J 2008;84:127–32.
72. Transverse Myelitis Consortium Working, Group. Proposed diagnostic criteria and nosology of acute transverse myelitis. Neurology 2002;59:499–505.
73. Goh C, Desmond PM, Phal PM. MRI in transverse myelitis. J Magn Reson Imaging 2014;40:1267–79.
74. Birnbaum J, Petri M, Thompson R, et al. Distinct subtypes of myelitis in systemic lupus erythematosus. Arthritis Rheum 2009;60:3378–87.
75. Fryer JP, Lennon VA, Pittock SJ, et al. AQP4 autoantibody assay performance in clinical laboratory service. Neurol Neuroimmunol Neuroinflamm 2014;1:e11.
76. West TW. Transverse myelitis–a review of the presentation, diagnosis, and initial management. Discov Med 2013;16:167–77.
77. Kitley JL, Leite MI, George JS, et al. The differential diagnosis of longitudinally extensive transverse myelitis. Mult Scler 2012;18:271–85.

78. Collongues N, de Seze J. An update on the evidence for the efficacy and safety of rituximab in the management of neuromyelitis optica. Ther Adv Neurol Disord 2016;9:180–8.
79. Kim SH, Huh SY, Lee SJ, et al. A 5-year follow-up of rituximab treatment in patients with neuromyelitis optica spectrum disorder. JAMA Neurol 2013;70:1110–7.
80. Kim SH, Kim W, Li XF, et al. Repeated treatment with rituximab based on the assessment of peripheral circulating memory B cells in patients with relapsing neuromyelitis optica over 2 years. Arch Neurol 2011;68:1412–20.
81. Govoni M, Bortoluzzi A, Padovan M, et al. The diagnosis and clinical management of the neuropsychiatric manifestations of lupus. J Autoimmun 2016;74: 41–72.
82. Magro-Checa C, Zirkzee EJ, Huizinga TW, et al. Management of neuropsychiatric systemic lupus erythematosus: current approaches and future perspectives. Drugs 2016;76:459–83.
83. Abbott NJ, Mendonca LL, Dolman DE. The blood-brain barrier in systemic lupus erythematosus. Lupus 2003;12:908–15.
84. Hanly JG. Avoiding diagnostic pitfalls in neuropsychiatric lupus: the importance of attribution. Lupus 2017;26:497–503.
85. Bortoluzzi A, Scire CA, Bombardieri S, et al. Development and validation of a new algorithm for attribution of neuropsychiatric events in systemic lupus erythematosus. Rheumatology (Oxford) 2015;54:891–8.
86. Magro-Checa C, Zirkzee EJ, Beaart-van de Voorde LJ, et al. Value of multidisciplinary reassessment in attribution of neuropsychiatric events to systemic lupus erythematosus: prospective data from the Leiden NPSLE cohort. Rheumatology (Oxford) 2017. [Epub ahead of print].
87. Pego-Reigosa JM, Cobo-Ibanez T, Calvo-Alen J, et al. Efficacy and safety of nonbiologic immunosuppressants in the treatment of nonrenal systemic lupus erythematosus: a systematic review. Arthritis Care Res (Hoboken) 2013;65:1775–85.
88. Barile-Fabris L, Ariza-Andraca R, Olguin-Ortega L, et al. Controlled clinical trial of IV cyclophosphamide versus IV methylprednisolone in severe neurological manifestations in systemic lupus erythematosus. Ann Rheum Dis 2005;64:620–5.
89. Fernandes Moca Trevisani V, Castro AA, Ferreira Neves Neto J, et al. Cyclophosphamide versus methylprednisolone for treating neuropsychiatric involvement in systemic lupus erythematosus. Cochrane Database Syst Rev 2013;(2):CD002265.
90. Cobo-Ibanez T, Loza-Santamaria E, Pego-Reigosa JM, et al. Efficacy and safety of rituximab in the treatment of non-renal systemic lupus erythematosus: a systematic review. Semin Arthritis Rheum 2014;44:175–85.
91. Tunnicliffe DJ, Singh-Grewal D, Kim S, et al. Diagnosis, monitoring, and treatment of systemic lupus erythematosus: a systematic review of clinical practice guidelines. Arthritis Care Res (Hoboken) 2015;67:1440–52.
92. Hanly JG, Urowitz MB, Su L, et al. Prospective analysis of neuropsychiatric events in an international disease inception cohort of patients with systemic lupus erythematosus. Ann Rheum Dis 2010;69:529–35.
93. Hanly JG, Urowitz MB, Su L, et al. Short-term outcome of neuropsychiatric events in systemic lupus erythematosus upon enrollment into an international inception cohort study. Arthritis Rheum 2008;59:721–9.
94. Hanly JG, Urowitz MB, Sanchez-Guerrero J, et al. Neuropsychiatric events at the time of diagnosis of systemic lupus erythematosus: an international inception cohort study. Arthritis Rheum 2007;56:265–73.

Central Nervous System Manifestations of Antiphospholipid Syndrome

Jonathan Graf, MD

KEYWORDS

- Antiphospholipid syndrome (APS) • Central nervous system (CNS) • Stroke • Chorea
- Psychosis • Cognitive disorder • Seizure • Sinus thrombosis

KEY POINTS

- Neurologic involvement is common in patients with antiphospholipid antibody syndrome.
- The most prevalent central nervous system manifestation of antiphospholipid syndrome is stroke, and the cerebral vasculature is the most commonly involved arterial bed in the body.
- Other thrombotic and nonthrombotic manifestations also have been reported that include cognitive disorders, dementia, seizures, chorea, migraine, psychosis, and demyelinating disease.
- In addition to infarction, neuroimaging often reveals white matter lesions throughout the brain that are nonspecific and also are seen in other conditions.
- Treatment of antiphospholipid antibody–associated neurologic disease consists of anticoagulation with or without additional immunosuppression as deemed necessary. The intensity of anticoagulation is a matter of some debate.

INTRODUCTION

The antiphospholipid syndrome (APS) is an acquired systemic disorder associated with circulating autoantibodies to anionic phospholipids and phospholipid binding complexes.[1] APS can occur independently (referred to as "primary APS") or in the setting of another autoimmune disease, most commonly systemic lupus erythematosus (SLE). The primary clinical manifestation of APS is thrombosis, which can occur in either the arterial or the venous circulation, or both. Neurologic involvement is prevalent in APS and responsible for significant morbidity and mortality from the disease.[2] APS affects the nervous system in myriad ways, with stroke and transient ischemic

Disclosure Statement: No disclosures.
Division of Rheumatology, University of California, Zuckerberg San Francisco General Hospital, San Francisco, 1001 Potrero Avenue, Box 0811, San Francisco, CA 94110, USA
E-mail address: Jonathan.Graf@ucsf.edu

Rheum Dis Clin N Am 43 (2017) 547–560
http://dx.doi.org/10.1016/j.rdc.2017.06.004
0889-857X/17/© 2017 Elsevier Inc. All rights reserved.

rheumatic.theclinics.com

attack (TIA) being the most common.[3] Not all neurologic manifestations, however, are a consequence of thrombotic events. This article reviews many neurologic complications (**Box 1**) linked to APS and focuses primarily on those that affect the central nervous system (CNS), reviewing their clinical features, diagnostic evaluation, and treatment.

CLINICAL MANIFESTATIONS
Cerebral Vascular Accident

The neurologic manifestations of APS can generally be grouped into those that are caused by ischemia and those that are not ischemia-related, with the former being more prevalent than the latter. Cerebrovascular accident (CVA) is the most common and often consequential neurologic complication of APS,[2] and the cerebral circulation is the most common arterial system affected in APS.[4] CVAs linked to APS can be either thrombotic or embolic in origin and can affect any vascular territory.[5] Antiphospholipid antibody (APL)-positive patients with ischemic stroke tend to be younger and more likely to be female compared with stroke patients who are APL negative.[6,7] Indeed, the prevalence of APS is particularly high in younger stroke patients. At least 20% of strokes in individuals younger than 45 are attributable to APS,[8] and the presence of APL in younger individuals confers a more than fivefold risk of incident stroke or TIA compared with those who are not APL positive.[9] Conversely, the risk of incident stroke associated with APL in older patients is somewhat less clear, and, although most studies that have examined this question support an increased risk of CVA in older patients who are APL positive,[5] the mechanism of APS-associated stroke may be different in younger patients than in older patients.[5] For those patients who have already suffered a CVA, there is some controversy as to whether the presence of APL increases the risk of a subsequent cerebral ischemic event.[2]

Patients with secondary APS in the setting of SLE also may be at greater risk of having a cerebral ischemic event than those with primary APS.[7] In this population, the presence of lupus anticoagulant (LAC) has been shown to be a stronger predictor of thrombosis and intracranial ischemic events than are antibodies to cardiolipin.[6,7,10] Traditional cardiovascular risk factors, such as hypertension, also have

---

Box 1
Central nervous system manifestations of antiphospholipid syndrome

Cerebral vascular accident

Sneddon syndrome

Venous sinus thrombosis

Cognitive impairment and dementia

Psychosis

Seizure

Movement disorder

Headache (including migraine)

Demyelinating disease

Transverse myelitis

Ischemic optic neuropathy

been linked to a greater risk for arterial thrombotic events and stroke in the setting of APS.[11]

A rare subset of patients with APS with stroke, particularly those with multiple smaller lacunar-type events, may actually have Sneddon syndrome, an independent entity that includes the presence of multiple cerebral infarctions and livedo reticularis. Whether Sneddon syndrome is a truly unique disease or merely a subclassification of APS is a matter of controversy. Up to 40% of patients with Sneddon syndrome have been found to be APL positive,[12] and clinical features such as livedo reticularis also have been reported in patients with APS. However, most patients with Sneddon syndrome are APL negative even on repeat testing, and clinical features such as livedo reticularis also can be seen in other disorders associated with ischemia of small dermal vessels. Patients with Sneddon syndrome generally fare worse and more often present with small vessel ischemia leading to significant cognitive deterioration and ischemic demyelination.[2]

In patients with APS, embolic strokes often originate from abnormalities of the cardiac valves.[2] Such valvular abnormalities are prevalent in up to one-third of patients who are APL positive, at least when visualized by transthoracic echocardiography.[13] The mitral valve is most commonly affected, followed by the aortic valve; lesions vary from thickening of the leaflets to frank, sterile endocarditis composed of platelets and fibrin.[2]

The clinical appearance of APS-associated ischemic stroke is generally similar to stroke that is not associated with APS.[4] The specific clinical manifestations of a stroke depend on the location and size of the occluded vessel.[2] Infarcts may be cortical, subcortical, or deep and affect any size vessel from small to large.[4] In the setting of a large-vessel infarct, angiography may identify an occlusion or stenosis, but often angiographic results will be relatively normal in the setting of transient neurologic compromise or with involvement of smaller-caliber vessels.[4] Multiple ischemic events involving small vessels may not present with overt sensory or motor deficits but rather with more subtle cognitive decline and dementia.

Cognitive Impairment and Dementia

Cognitive impairment and dementia are frequently reported in patients with APS.[14] Although age and presence of livedo reticularis may correlate with cognitive decline, the correlation between stroke and cognitive impairment in patients with APS has not been as well studied.[15,16] Several studies of patients with and without SLE have demonstrated a positive relationship between cognitive dysfunction and both anticardiolipin antibody titer and persistence.[5,17-19] In one study, one-third of nonelderly patients with asymptomatic APL were found to have cognitive deficits.[17] Among patients who meet criteria for APS, the prevalence of global cognitive impairment may be 42% or even higher, and formal neuropsychiatric testing can often detect abnormalities of complex attention, verbal learning and fluency, visuospatial ability, executive functioning, and memory.[14,15,17,20] This appears to correlate with functional MRI, as demonstrated in a pilot study that showed abnormal brain activity particularly in the frontal lobes of patients with APS who were examined during executive functioning and memory tasks.[21] Although MRI in some studies of patients with APS with neurologic symptoms demonstrated a high frequency of cortical, subcortical, and basal ganglia infarcts (many of which are silent), other studies focusing specifically on cognition did not show increased numbers of infarcts in patients with APS with cognitive deficits compared with those without.[15,16,22] MRI of patients with APS with cognitive deficits often reveals increased numbers of white matter lesions compared with those without such deficits.[15] The appearance of these lesions varies in appearance from small and focal to more diffuse in nature, but whether these lesions represent ischemic or inflammatory demyelinating processes is not always clear.[16,22]

Dementia is reported less frequently in association with APS than is cognitive dysfunction. The frequency of dementia in patients with APS has been reported to be anywhere from 0% to 6%, including a reported frequency of 2.5% in a well-characterized cohort of 1000 patients with APS.[14,23] Among elderly patients, however, the prevalence of dementia may be higher, as suggested in a study of 23 patients with APS with a mean age of 65 that found a frequency of 56% when dementia was defined using standard psychiatric criteria.[16,24] Although the association between APS and dementia is thought to be primarily related to multiple small vessel infarctions in a manner similar to what is observed in patients with multi-infarct dementia,[4] case reports of dementia and other features of APS that reverse with immunosuppression suggest that alternative mechanisms may drive dementia development in at least some patients.[25]

Venous Sinus Thrombosis

APS is not only implicated in thrombosis of the arterial circulation of the CNS but also in cerebral venous sinus thrombosis. Although a relatively rare phenomenon, venous sinus thrombosis has been linked to the presence of anticardiolipin and other APL antibodies and is generally more prevalent in younger individuals, with more extensive superficial and deep involvement than in dural venous thrombosis that is not associated with APS. Clinically, venous sinus thrombosis presents with more protean symptoms, such as refractory headache, but can evolve to cause intracranial hypertension, seizures, and focal neurologic deficits.[7] There is often a delay in diagnosis, and some patients can initially present with transient and stuttering neurologic deficits with unremarkable computed tomography imaging.[26] Earlier treatment portends a better prognosis.[7]

Seizures and Epilepsy

The prevalence of seizure disorder in patients with APS has been reported to be between 7.0% and 8.6% in some studies.[27,28] The prevalence may be higher in patients with secondary APS, in whom the frequency of epilepsy has been reported to be 13.7%.[28] Similarly in patients with SLE, the frequency of seizures is higher in those who are APL positive compared with those without APL.[29–31] This association appears to be stronger in patients who have higher-titer, immunoglobulin (Ig)G anticardiolipin antibodies than in those with lower-titer IgM antibodies.[30] The use of antiepileptic drugs to treat seizures complicates these analyses somewhat, as these medications have been implicated in inducing APL. In one prospective study, APL was detected in 43% of patients with seizure treated with antiepileptic medications such as phenytoin and valproate; however, most of these patients had IgM-specific anticardiolipin antibodies.[32,33] Another study of newly diagnosed patients with epilepsy who were not yet taking antiepileptic drugs found a higher prevalence of IgG anticardiolipin antibodies compared with controls, suggesting that the link between these antibodies and seizures persists even in the absence of these medications.[34]

In most cases, APL likely induces seizures by causing ischemic damage to brain parenchyma and generating epileptogenic foci.[14] Thromboembolic CNS events constituted the largest risk factor for development of epilepsy in a cohort of more than 500 patients with APS, with an odds ratio of more than 4:1.[28] Other ischemia-related risk factors associated with seizure development include livedo reticularis, smoking, and valvular heart disease.[14,28,35] Despite the prominent role that APL-mediated ischemia plays in the development of epilepsy, not every case appears to be ischemia-driven. A study examining the prevalence of APL in 3 distinct cohorts of patients with seizure demonstrated a higher frequency of APL in patients compared with controls, yet none of these patients had ischemic or thrombotic lesions on neuro-imaging.[33,34] APL has been shown to bind directly to ependymal, myelin, and other brain tissue, suggesting a potential immunologic basis for APL-mediated epilepsy.[5] One study has shown that IgG from patients with high APL titers depolarizes brain synaptoneurosomes from rats, whereas another has demonstrated that APL obtained from patients with SLE patients with seizures reduces a gamma-aminobutyric acid receptor–mediated chloride current in snail neurons.[5,36]

Chorea

Chorea is the most common movement disorder associated with APS (primary APS as well as APS with SLE).[4,14] Its prevalence in APS ranges between 1.3% and 4.5%.[17,27,37] Other reported movement disorders include ballismus, dyskinesia, parkinsonism, and cerebellar ataxia.[14] Chorea can be either generalized or involve only one side of the body and can evolve over several weeks or, in some cases, even longer.[4] Many of these patients are young, female, and have secondary or SLE-associated APS.[38] One possible trigger for chorea in these patients may be the introduction of oral contraception.[38] Although clinical correlation between APL and chorea appears to be fairly well established, the pathophysiological basis for the disorder is not well understood but may involve direct antibody-mediated effects on the basal ganglia.[39] In other instances, ischemic insults to the caudate or putamen or both also may play a role.[4] Treatment involves symptomatic relief with dopamine receptor antagonists, but often chorea responds well to immunosuppression with corticosteroids and cyclophosphamide.[4]

Headache and Migraine

Chronic headache and migraine are commonly observed in patients with APS. In one study of 1000 patients, 202 patients (20.2%) experienced migraine headaches.[27] Because headache is so common in the general population, it is not surprising that some studies have failed to show an increased prevalence of APL in patients with migraine, either with or without SLE.[40] Nevertheless, migraine in patients with APS can be a harbinger of more severe ischemic disease to follow. A review of 162 consecutive patients with stoke identified 10 patients who were APL positive, with 6 of these having experienced a long-standing history of migraine headaches compared with only 5 of 152 patients with stroke who were APL negative.[41] Migraine headaches associated with APS may be difficult to control with typical analgesic regimens and persist for years before patients are recognized as having APS.[2,42] One investigator reported significant clinical improvement in headaches after anticoagulant therapy, suggesting not only a possible role of APL-mediated ischemia but also providing an argument for screening for APL in patients with particularly difficult and refractory migraines.[8]

Multiple Sclerosis–like Disease

APS has been linked to multiple sclerosis (MS)-type lesions, ischemic optic neuropathy, and transverse myelitis. These entities can be difficult to distinguish from their idiopathic counterparts, in part because there are no definitive tests to distinguish between either MS or APS. Testing for oligoclonal bands in the cerebral spinal fluid or APL in the serum is not specific for either MS or APL, respectively.[2] One study prospectively examined patients with presumed MS and found no clinical differences between patients with MS with or without APL.[43] Another examined 20 of 100 patients with MS who were APL positive and found atypical clinical features, including a slower progression of myelopathy and clinical deterioration, a higher prevalence of headache, and a lower prevalence of oligoclonal bands in the cerebral spinal fluid[44]; 30% of these patients also had optic neuropathy.[44] There have been some reports of good responses to anticoagulant therapy in these patients, suggesting that although APS-associated MS and its idiopathic counterpart may be difficult to distinguish from one another, the mechanisms underlying these 2 disorders may be quite different.[45]

Transverse myelitis is a rare event, even in patients with SLE in whom its prevalence is reported to be less than 1%.[5] It presents with acute or subacute onset of a sensory-level deficit, paraparesis or quadriparesis, and bowel or bladder dysfunction and usually affects the thoracic segment of the spinal cord.[4,46] Interestingly, one study of 14 patients with SLE and transverse myelitis and an additional review of 91 cases in the literature found 43% and 64%, respectively, were APL positive, suggesting a strong association between transverse myelitis and APL in patients with SLE.[47] Most patients respond to pulse corticosteroid therapy with or without anticoagulation, and other patients have also demonstrated further responses to cyclophosphamide treatment.[4,48]

Neuropsychiatric Disease

An increased prevalence of APL has been reported in patients with psychosis. Many antipsychotic medications have themselves also been linked to APL, usually IgM-specific cardiolipin or LAC antibodies.[49] One study examined 34 acutely psychotic patients before receiving any antipsychotic medications and found that 32% of them were positive for APL (more often IgG-cardiolipin antibodies than LAC) compared with none of their healthy controls.[49] By entry criteria, none of these study patients were permitted to have evidence of SLE, other autoimmune-related disorders, or other clinical features of APS (history of thrombosis, other vascular events, or fetal loss).[49] Another study examined 100 patients admitted to the hospital with hallucinations or delusions or both and found that 25% of patients were positive for APL using expanded testing for antibodies directed against not only IgG, IgM, and IgA isotypes of cardiolipin but also against phosphatidylethanolamine, phosphatidylserine, and phosphatidylcholine.[50] Patients with chronic schizophrenia also have increased frequency of APL, and case reports have detailed episodes of other axis I disorders in patients with APL that include bipolar and obsessive compulsive disorders.[14,50–52] Those patients who are older, have a history of cerebral ischemia, or are triple antibody positive (anticardiolipin, anti–beta-2-glycoprotein 1 [B2GP1], and LAC) appear to be at greatest risk for neuropsychiatric disease.[14]

CLASSIFICATION CRITERIA, LABORATORY, AND IMAGING FINDINGS
Classification Criteria for Antiphospholipid Syndrome and Laboratory Testing

International working groups have established criteria for the classification of patients with APS (**Box 2**).[53] Because these criteria have been optimized to facilitate studies of patients with APS, they sacrifice diagnostic sensitivity for specificity and do not necessarily identify all patients with clinical manifestations of the disease.[1] For example, for patients to be classified with APS by the most recent criteria, they must experience an arterial or venous thrombosis or pregnancy morbidity and also have a positive test for APL on 2 occasions no fewer than 12 weeks and no more than 5 years apart.[53] Although APS can affect the CNS in multiple ways, only stoke and TIA fall within the spectrum of thrombotic disease included in the formal classification criteria. Other well-recognized symptoms, such as cognitive dysfunction, headache or migraine, MS, transverse myelopathy, or epilepsy are not recognized in the criteria.[53]

> **Box 2**
> **Classification criteria for antiphospholipid syndrome**
>
> *Clinical Criteria (at least 1 of the following):*
>
> 1. Vascular thrombosis
>   One or more clinical episodes of arterial, venous, or small vessel thrombosis, in any tissue or organ.
>
> 2. Pregnancy morbidity
>   - One or more unexplained deaths of a morphologically normal fetus at or beyond the 10th week of gestation
>   - One or more premature births of a morphologically normal neonate before the 34th week of gestation because of eclampsia or severe preeclampsia (placental insufficiency)
>   - Three or more unexplained consecutive spontaneous abortions before the 10th week of gestation
>
> *Laboratory Criteria (at least 1)*
>
> 1. Anticardiolipin antibody
>   Immunoglobulin (Ig)G and/or IgM isotype in medium or high titer (>40 GPL) on 2 or more occasions, at least 12 weeks apart
>
> 2. Anti–beta-2-glycoprotein-I antibody
>   IgG and/or IgM (in titer >the 99th percentile), present on 2 or more occasions, at least 12 weeks apart
>
> 3. Lupus anticoagulant
>   Present in plasma, on 2 or more occasions at least 12 weeks apart
>
> *Adapted from* Miyakis S, Lockshin MD, Atsumi T, et al. International consensus statement on an update of the classification criteria for definite antiphospholipid syndrome (APS). J Thromb Haemost 2006;4(2):295–306.

Nevertheless, the consensus statement does recognize these sequelae as neurologic-specific manifestations of APS in the appropriate clinical context.[53] Similarly, the criteria's requirement for a second confirmatory APL test at least 12 weeks after the first is not always a practical one, as clinical circumstances may warrant treating patients with anticoagulant agents before obtaining the second test, a reality that can complicate interpretation of LAC testing.[1]

According to current APS classification criteria, patients with APS must demonstrate moderate to high titers of antibodies as detected by at least 1 of 3 types of tests: (1) solid-phase immunoassays for antibodies to cardiolipin, (2) solid-phase immunoassays for antibodies to B2GP1, and/or (3) functional testing for inhibitors that have LAC activity.[53] All 3 tests should be used when evaluating a patient with suspected APS. The classification criteria do not formally recognize positive testing for IgA anticardiolipin antibodies nor do they address patients who test positive for antibodies to phosphatidylethanolamine, phosphatidylserine, and phosphatidylcholine in extended phospholipid antibody panels, because these tests are judged to lack specificity. However, this does not completely exclude patients from a diagnosis of APS if they test positive only for these types of antibodies.

Anticardiolipin antibodies recognize epitopes on cardiolipin, an anionic phospholipid that is a component of the inner membrane of mitochondria, and the risk of thrombosis has been shown to correlate both with IgG isotype and titer. Of the 3 types of APL tests, anticardiolipin antibody testing is most sensitive but least specific for APS, in part because these antibodies are often transiently and asymptomatically induced by various medications as well as acute and chronic infections.[54] Antibodies to B2Gp1 recognize epitopes on the phospholipid binding protein itself or on the macromolecular complex created by binding between B2Gp1 and cardiolipin. These antibodies are more specifically associated with APS and thrombotic events than are antibodies that bind only to cardiolipin.[54]

LAC activity refers to a family of antibodies that collectively demonstrate the ability to prolong in vitro phospholipid-dependent clotting assays. The target antigen(s) of these antibodies are not formally determined in LAC testing. Rather, their presence is deduced from a multistep process that generally includes (1) demonstrating prolongation of an in vitro coagulation test, (2) demonstrating with a mixing study that the prolongation is due to an inhibitor and not to a factor deficiency, and (3) demonstrating the phospholipid-dependence of the inhibitor by correcting the prolonged clotting time with addition of excess phospholipid reagent. Antibodies to cardiolipin and B2GP1 often but not always have LAC activity. Conversely, many patients with APS have LAC but not antibodies to either cardiolipin or B2GP1. The functional testing required to detect LAC can be labor intensive and tedious.[54] Furthermore, there are several different assays commonly used to detect LAC (**Table 1**), with each having its own unique testing characteristics. Thus, there is generally less standardization in performance and testing for LAC than there is for testing of anticardiolipin or anti-B2GP1 antibodies. If the index of suspicion remains high for a patient with suspected APS, testing for LAC should be repeated with at least one different method.[54] LAC antibodies have more specificity but less sensitivity for APS and thus have been shown to correlate more strongly with risk of thrombosis than antibodies to either cardiolipin or B2GP1.[54]

Neuroimaging

Patients with APS often but not always demonstrate abnormalities on neuroimaging studies.[14] The most common of these are focal areas of signal hyperintensity scattered throughout the subcortical white matter.[5,22,55] Whether these lesions represent ischemia, inflammation, or both in each patient is not always clear.[22] White matter disease has been demonstrated both in patients with APS with focal neurologic deficits as well as in patients with more general neurologic manifestations such as seizure or cognitive dysfunction.[40,56] This pattern is generally nonspecific and can be seen in

Table 1	
Commonly used assays to detect lupus anticoagulant	
Test Name	**Test Description**
Activated partial thromboplastin time (aPTT)	Test of intrinsic clotting cascade requiring use of phospholipid reagents
Dilute aPTT	Enhanced sensitivity aPTT using limiting concentrations of phospholipid reagents
Dilute Russell viper venom time	Sensitive test that uses very small amounts of phospholipid reagents
Hexagonal phase phospholipid (HPE) neutralization	Ratio comparing 2 simultaneous PTTs performed with and without HPE reagent
Platelet neutralization test	Similar to HPE neutralization but uses platelet extracts in the confirmatory step

From Graf J. Chapter 23. Antiphospholipid antibody syndrome. In: Imboden JB, Hellmann DB, Stone JH, editors. Current diagnosis & treatment: rheumatology. New York: The McGraw-Hill Companies; 2013. Accessed May 21, 2017.

other disease processes.[5] In the setting of ischemic stroke, imaging will usually demonstrate clear areas of infarction, which can be small or large and involve both superficial and deeper areas of the brain.[4] Often, angiography will show large-vessel occlusion without evidence of vasculitis or be otherwise unremarkable.[57] Other case series have observed multiple infarcts and encephalomalacia on neuroimaging of young patients with APS presenting with neuropsychiatric disease, including depression, encephalopathy, and generalized movement disorder.[58]

Treatment

The treatment of patients with APS who present with neurologic disease depends on the specific manifestation, its severity, and its presumed underlying mechanism. Antithrombotic treatment serves as first-line therapy for patients whose symptoms are linked to thrombo-occlusive disease. Aspirin and newer antiplatelet agents, heparin, and warfarin have all served as cornerstones of antithrombotic treatment, but significant controversy remains regarding which specific agent and what intensity of therapy should be used.[2,7] Some investigators advocate use of aspirin for primary prevention in patients with persistently positive anticardiolipin antibodies or LAC.[5] For secondary prevention of recurrent thromboembolic event, most investigators recommend using an unfractionated or low molecular weight heparin bridge followed by standard-dose therapy with warfarin targeting an International Normalized Ratio (INR) range between 2 and 3.[2,5,59,60] Most of these recommendations are based on a prospective randomized trial of patients with APS assigned to standard-intensity and high-intensity warfarin regimens.[61] Although this trial failed to demonstrate a difference between these 2 groups in either recurrent thrombotic events or in bleeding complications, several important limitations of the trial should be considered, including the exclusion of patients with recurrent thrombosis or recent stroke and the fact that many patients assigned to intensive therapy remained below their target INR of 3 to 4.[7,61] Citing these concerns and belief that the danger of stoke outweighs the risk of bleeding, the European League Against Rheumatism has issued guidelines recommending the consideration of high-intensity warfarin therapy for patients with ischemic stroke in the setting of APS.[62]

There remains less evidence supporting the use of anticoagulation in patients with APS with neurologic symptoms not clearly explained by thrombosis. In some case reports, use of anticoagulation in patients with migraine, neuropsychiatric disease, and transverse myelitis has resulted in significant improvement in symptoms.[63–65] An international consensus has also recommended use of anticoagulation in patients with APL associated valvular heart disease who are at risk for thrombosis but did not endorse use of corticosteroids.[46,66] Finally, for cases of cognitive dysfunction, current European League Against Rheumatism guidelines suggest consideration of antiplatelet or anticoagulation therapy in patients with SLE, APL, and severe neuropsychiatric disease.[67]

Those patients who experience refractory thrombotic disease on standard-intensity warfarin can increase the intensity of their anticoagulation to target a higher INR in the range of 3 to 4.[46] For patients with APS who break through high-intensity therapy or for those presumed to have nonischemic neurologic disease, use of immunosuppressive therapy alone or in combination with anticoagulation has been used with some success.[68,69] Thus, some investigators recommend treating neurologic manifestations of APS that do not clearly appear to be ischemic in origin with a combination of antithrombotic therapy for at least 6 months plus corticosteroids and/or other immunosuppressive therapy.[46] Symptomatic treatment of chorea or psychosis with antidopaminergic therapy or epilepsy with anticonvulsants can be very effective as well.[46,67] Statin therapy also should be considered, particularly for patients who experience thrombotic disease.[7] When needed, the choice of immunosuppressive therapy will depend on the individual characteristics of a patient and his or her disease manifestation. Therapies including corticosteroids, mycophenolate mofetil, azathioprine, and cyclophosphamide have all been used, although data supporting their use has been mixed.[2,7,46] Hydroxychloroquine treatment may be particularly useful for secondary patients with APS with SLE.[7] For the most severe cases, treatment with intravenous gammaglobulin, plasmapheresis, and rituximab therapy also may be of benefit.[2,14]

REFERENCES

1. Graf J. Chapter 23. Antiphospholipid antibody syndrome. In: Imboden JB, Hellmann DB, Stone JH, editors. Current diagnosis & treatment: rheumatology. New York: The McGraw-Hill Companies; 2013. Available at: accessmedicine. mhmedical.com/content.aspx?aid=57272448. Accessed May 21, 2017.
2. Rodrigues CEM, Carvalho JF, Shoenfeld Y. Neurological manifestations of antiphospholipid syndrome. Eur J Clin Invest 2010;40(4):350–9.
3. Levine JS, Branch DW, Rauch J. The antiphospholipid syndrome. N Engl J Med 2002;346(10):752–63.
4. Tanne D, Hassin-Baer S. Neurologic manifestations of the antiphospholipid syndrome. Curr Rheumatol Rep 2001;3(4):286–92.
5. Roldan JF, Brey RL. Neurologic manifestations of the antiphospholipid syndrome. Curr Rheumatol Rep 2007;9(2):109–15.
6. Hanly JG, Urowitz MB, Su L, et al. Autoantibodies as biomarkers for the prediction of neuropsychiatric events in systemic lupus erythematosus. Ann Rheum Dis 2011;70(10):1726–32.
7. de Amorim LCD, Maia FM, Rodrigues CEM. Stroke in systemic lupus erythematosus and antiphospholipid syndrome: risk factors, clinical manifestations, neuroimaging, and treatment. Lupus 2017;26(5):529–36.
8. Hughes GRV. Migraine, memory loss, and "multiple sclerosis." Neurological features of the antiphospholipid (Hughes') syndrome. Postgrad Med J 2003;79(928): 81–3.
9. Sciascia S, Sanna G, Khamashta MA, et al. The estimated frequency of antiphospholipid antibodies in young adults with cerebrovascular events: a systematic review. Ann Rheum Dis 2015;74(11):2028–33.
10. Petri M, Rheinschmidt M, Whiting-O'Keefe Q, et al. The frequency of lupus anticoagulant in systemic lupus erythematosus. A study of sixty consecutive patients by activated partial thromboplastin time, Russell viper venom time, and anticardiolipin antibody level. Ann Intern Med 1987;106(4):524–31.
11. de Souza AWS, Silva NP, de Carvalho JF, et al. Impact of hypertension and hyperhomocysteinemia on arterial thrombosis in primary antiphospholipid syndrome. Lupus 2007;16(10):782–7.
12. Francès C, Papo T, Wechsler B, et al. Sneddon syndrome with or without antiphospholipid antibodies. A comparative study in 46 patients. Medicine (Baltimore) 1999;78(4):209–19.
13. Tenedios F, Erkan D, Lockshin MD. Cardiac manifestations in the antiphospholipid syndrome. Rheum Dis Clin North Am 2006;32(3):491–507.
14. Yelnik CM, Kozora E, Appenzeller S. Non-stroke central neurologic manifestations in antiphospholipid syndrome. Curr Rheumatol Rep 2016;18(2):11.

15. Tektonidou MG, Varsou N, Kotoulas G, et al. Cognitive deficits in patients with antiphospholipid syndrome: association with clinical, laboratory, and brain magnetic resonance imaging findings. Arch Intern Med 2006;166(20):2278–84.
16. Yelnik CM, Kozora E, Appenzeller S. Cognitive disorders and antiphospholipid antibodies. Autoimmun Rev 2016;15(12):1193–8.
17. Jacobson MW, Rapport LJ, Keenan PA, et al. Neuropsychological deficits associated with antiphospholipid antibodies. J Clin Exp Neuropsychol 1999;21(2):251–64.
18. Menon S, Jameson-Shortall E, Newman SP, et al. A longitudinal study of anticardiolipin antibody levels and cognitive functioning in systemic lupus erythematosus. Arthritis Rheum 1999;42(4):735–41.
19. Hanly JG, Hong C, Smith S, et al. A prospective analysis of cognitive function and anticardiolipin antibodies in systemic lupus erythematosus. Arthritis Rheum 1999;42(4):728–34.
20. Kozora E, Erkan D, Zhang L, et al. Cognitive dysfunction in antiphospholipid antibody (aPL)-negative systemic lupus erythematosus (SLE) versus aPL-positive non-SLE patients. Clin Exp Rheumatol 2014;32(1):34–40.
21. Kozora E, Uluğ AM, Erkan D, et al. Functional magnetic resonance imaging of working memory and executive dysfunction in systemic lupus erythematosus and antiphospholipid antibody-positive patients. Arthritis Care Res 2016;68(11):1655–63.
22. Zhu D-S, Fu J, Zhang Y, et al. Neurological antiphospholipid syndrome: clinical, neuroimaging, and pathological characteristics. J Neurol Sci 2014;346(1–2):138–44.
23. Cervera R, Piette J-C, Font J, et al. Antiphospholipid syndrome: clinical and immunologic manifestations and patterns of disease expression in a cohort of 1,000 patients. Arthritis Rheum 2002;46(4):1019–27.
24. Chapman J, Abu-Katash M, Inzelberg R, et al. Prevalence and clinical features of dementia associated with the antiphospholipid syndrome and circulating anticoagulants. J Neurol Sci 2002;203–204:81–4.
25. Van Horn G, Arnett FC, Dimachkie MM. Reversible dementia and chorea in a young woman with the lupus anticoagulant. Neurology 1996;46(6):1599–603.
26. Tsai C-L, Hueng D-Y, Tsao W-L, et al. Cerebral venous sinus thrombosis as an initial manifestation of primary antiphospholipid syndrome. Am J Emerg Med 2013;31(5):888.e1-3.
27. Cervera R, Boffa M-C, Khamashta MA, et al. The Euro-Phospholipid project: epidemiology of the antiphospholipid syndrome in Europe. Lupus 2009;18(10):889–93.
28. Shoenfeld Y, Lev S, Blatt I, et al. Features associated with epilepsy in the antiphospholipid syndrome. J Rheumatol 2004;31(7):1344–8.
29. Herranz MT, Rivier G, Khamashta MA, et al. Association between antiphospholipid antibodies and epilepsy in patients with systemic lupus erythematosus. Arthritis Rheum 1994;37(4):568–71.
30. Cimaz R, Meroni PL, Shoenfeld Y. Epilepsy as part of systemic lupus erythematosus and systemic antiphospholipid syndrome (Hughes syndrome). Lupus 2006;15(4):191–7.
31. Appenzeller S, Condea Γ, Costallal LTL. Epileptic seizures in systemic lupus erythematosus. Neurology 2004;63(10):1808–12.
32. Pardo A, González-Porque P, Gobernado JM, et al. Study of antiphospholipid antibodies in patients treated with antiepileptic drugs. Neurologica 2001;16(1):7–10.

33. Chapman J, Rand JH, Brey RL, et al. Non-stroke neurological syndromes associated with antiphospholipid antibodies: evaluation of clinical and experimental studies. Lupus 2003;12(7):514–7.

34. Peltola JT, Haapala A, Isojärvi JI, et al. Antiphospholipid and antinuclear antibodies in patients with epilepsy or new-onset seizure disorders. Am J Med 2000;109(9):712–7.

35. de Carvalho JF, Pasoto SG, Appenzeller S. Seizures in primary antiphospholipid syndrome: the relevance of smoking to stroke. Clin Dev Immunol 2012;2012: 981519.

36. Chapman J, Cohen-Armon M, Shoenfeld Y, et al. Antiphospholipid antibodies permeabilize and depolarize brain synaptoneurosomes. Lupus 1999;8(2): 127–33.

37. Appenzeller S, Yeh S, Maruyama M, et al. Chorea in primary antiphospholipid syndrome is associated with rheumatic fever. Rheumatol Int 2012;32(9):2857–61.

38. Cervera R, Asherson RA, Font J, et al. Chorea in the antiphospholipid syndrome. Clinical, radiologic, and immunologic characteristics of 50 patients from our clinics and the recent literature. Medicine (Baltimore) 1997;76(3):203–12.

39. Katzav A, Chapman J, Shoenfeld Y. CNS dysfunction in the antiphospholipid syndrome. Lupus 2003;12(12):903–7.

40. Tietjen GE, Day M, Norris L, et al. Role of anticardiolipin antibodies in young persons with migraine and transient focal neurologic events: a prospective study. Neurology 1998;50(5):1433–40.

41. Silvestrini M, Cupini LM, Matteis M, et al. Migraine in patients with stroke and antiphospholipid antibodies. Headache 1993;33(8):421–6.

42. Sanna G, D'Cruz D, Cuadrado MJ. Cerebral manifestations in the antiphospholipid (Hughes) syndrome. Rheum Dis Clin North Am 2006;32(3):465–90.

43. Tourbah A, Clapin A, Gout O, et al. Systemic autoimmune features and multiple sclerosis: a 5-year follow-up study. Arch Neurol 1998;55(4):517–21.

44. Karussis D, Leker RR, Ashkenazi A, et al. A subgroup of multiple sclerosis patients with anticardiolipin antibodies and unusual clinical manifestations: do they represent a new nosological entity? Ann Neurol 1998;44(4):629–34.

45. Cuadrado MJ, Khamashta MA, Ballesteros A, et al. Can neurologic manifestations of Hughes (antiphospholipid) syndrome be distinguished from multiple sclerosis? Analysis of 27 patients and review of the literature. Medicine (Baltimore) 2000;79(1):57–68.

46. Espinosa G, Cervera R. Current treatment of antiphospholipid syndrome: lights and shadows. Nat Rev Rheumatol 2015;11(10):586–96.

47. Kovacs B, Lafferty TL, Brent LH, et al. Transverse myelopathy in systemic lupus erythematosus: an analysis of 14 cases and review of the literature. Ann Rheum Dis 2000;59(2):120–4.

48. Aziz A, Conway MD, Robertson HJ, et al. Acute optic neuropathy and transverse myelopathy in patients with antiphospholipid antibody syndrome: favorable outcome after treatment with anticoagulants and glucocorticoids. Lupus 2000; 9(4):307–10.

49. Schwartz M, Rochas M, Weller B, et al. High association of anticardiolipin antibodies with psychosis. J Clin Psychiatry 1998;59(1):20–3.

50. Sokol DK, O'Brien RS, Wagenknecht DR, et al. Antiphospholipid antibodies in blood and cerebrospinal fluids of patients with psychosis. J Neuroimmunol 2007;190(1–2):151–6.

51. Chengappa KN, Carpenter AB, Keshavan MS, et al. Elevated IGG and IGM anti-cardiolipin antibodies in a subgroup of medicated and unmedicated schizophrenic patients. Biol Psychiatry 1991;30(7):731–5.

52. Avari JN, Young RC. A patient with bipolar disorder and antiphospholipid syndrome. J Geriatr Psychiatry Neurol 2012;25(1):26–8.

53. Miyakis S, Lockshin MD, Atsumi T, et al. International consensus statement on an update of the classification criteria for definite antiphospholipid syndrome (APS). J Thromb Haemost 2006;4(2):295–306.

54. Bertolaccini ML, Khamashta MA. Laboratory diagnosis and management challenges in the antiphospholipid syndrome. Lupus 2006;15(3):172–8.

55. Erkan D, Kozora E, Lockshin MD. Cognitive dysfunction and white matter abnormalities in antiphospholipid syndrome. Pathophysiology 2011;18(1):93–102.

56. Toubi E, Khamashta MA, Panarra A, et al. Association of antiphospholipid antibodies with central nervous system disease in systemic lupus erythematosus. Am J Med 1995;99(4):397–401.

57. Levine SR, Deegan MJ, Futrell N, et al. Cerebrovascular and neurologic disease associated with antiphospholipid antibodies: 48 cases. Neurology 1990;40(8):1181–9.

58. Li C-H, Chou M-C, Liu C-K, et al. Antiphospholipid syndrome presenting as progressive neuropsychiatric disorders: two case reports. Neuropsychiatr Dis Treat 2013;9:739–42.

59. Marshall AL, Connors J-M. Anticoagulation for noncardiac indications in neurologic patients: comparative use of non-vitamin K oral anticoagulants, low-molecular-weight heparins, and warfarin. Curr Treat Options Neurol 2014;16(9):309.

60. Lim W, Crowther MA, Eikelboom JW. Management of antiphospholipid antibody syndrome: a systematic review. JAMA 2006;295(9):1050–7.

61. Crowther MA, Ginsberg JS, Julian J, et al. A comparison of two intensities of warfarin for the prevention of recurrent thrombosis in patients with the antiphospholipid antibody syndrome. N Engl J Med 2003;349(12):1133–8.

62. Bertsias G, Ioannidis JPA, Boletis J, et al. EULAR recommendations for the management of systemic lupus erythematosus. Report of a Task Force of the EULAR Standing Committee for International Clinical Studies Including Therapeutics. Ann Rheum Dis 2008;67(2):195–205.

63. Asherson RA, Giampaulo D, Singh S, et al. Dramatic response of severe headaches to anticoagulation in a patient with antiphospholipid syndrome. J Clin Rheumatol 2007;13(3):173–4.

64. Roie EV, Labarque V, Renard M, et al. Obsessive-compulsive behavior as presenting symptom of primary antiphospholipid syndrome. Psychosom Med 2013;75(3):326–30.

65. D'Cruz DP, Mellor-Pita S, Joven B, et al. Transverse myelitis as the first manifestation of systemic lupus erythematosus or lupus-like disease: good functional outcome and relevance of antiphospholipid antibodies. J Rheumatol 2004;31(2):280–5.

66. Lockshin M, Tenedios F, Petri M, et al. Cardiac disease in the antiphospholipid syndrome: recommendations for treatment. Committee consensus report. Lupus 2003;12(7):518–23.

67. Bertsias GK, Ioannidis JPA, Aringer M, et al. EULAR recommendations for the management of systemic lupus erythematosus with neuropsychiatric manifestations: report of a task force of the EULAR standing committee for clinical affairs. Ann Rheum Dis 2010;69(12):2074–82.

68. Carecchio M, Comi C, Varrasi C, et al. Complex movement disorders in primary antiphospholipid syndrome: a case report. J Neurol Sci 2009;281(1–2):101–3.

69. Lai J-Y, Wu P-C, Chen H-C, et al. Early neuropsychiatric involvement in antiphospholipid syndrome. Gen Hosp Psychiatry 2012;34(5):579.e1-3.

Neurologic Manifestations of Rheumatoid Arthritis

Kimberly DeQuattro, MD, John B. Imboden, MD*

KEYWORDS

- Rheumatoid arthritis • Atlantoaxial subluxation • Cervical spine subluxation
- Rheumatoid meningitis • Rheumatoid vasculitis • Compression neuropathy

KEY POINTS

- Aggressive medical management of rheumatoid arthritis can prevent the development cervical spine disease but does not halt progression of preexisting cervical lesions.
- MRI is the imaging modality of choice for the assessment of the rheumatoid patient with neurologic symptoms or signs attributable to cervical spine disease.
- Myelopathy due to rheumatoid cervical spine disease is progressive and requires surgical intervention.
- Rheumatoid meningitis is rare but should be considered when a patient with long-standing rheumatoid arthritis develops new neurologic findings that point to an intracranial process.
- Compressive neuropathy, particularly carpal tunnel syndrome, is the most common abnormality of the peripheral nervous system in rheumatoid arthritis.

INVOLVEMENT OF THE CERVICAL SPINE
Overview

Involvement of the cervical spine is common in rheumatoid arthritis (RA) (approaching 80% in some studies) and ranges in severity from an asymptomatic radiographic abnormality to a life-threatening condition.[1,2] RA can affect the atlantooccipital joint (C1-occiput), the atlantoaxial joint (C1-C2), and the subaxial joints (C3-C7). As is the case with peripheral joint disease in RA, inflammation of the synovial-lined joints of the cervical spine leads to pannus formation and erosion of juxta-articular bone, thereby damaging articular structures and weakening adjacent ligaments.[3] Although inflammatory lesions can directly compress the spinal cord and nerve roots, most

Supported by the Arthritis Foundation and by the Russell Engleman Rheumatology Research Center.

Drs K. DeQuattro and J.B. Imboden have no financial disclosures and no conflicts of interest.

Division of Rheumatology, Department of Medicine, University of California, San Francisco, San Francisco, CA, USA

* Corresponding author. University of California, San Francisco, Box 0868, San Francisco, CA 94143.

E-mail address: john.imboden@ucsf.edu

Rheum Dis Clin N Am 43 (2017) 561–571
http://dx.doi.org/10.1016/j.rdc.2017.06.005
0889-857X/17/© 2017 Elsevier Inc. All rights reserved.

rheumatic.theclinics.com

serious complications stem from structural alterations of the cervical spine, particularly subluxations of the atlantoaxial and atlantooccipital joints, which can lead to compression of the spinal cord, impingement of the brainstem, compromise of the vertebral arteries, and impingement of spinal nerve roots or cranial nerves. Destabilization of the lower cervical spine due to extension of inflammation into the discovertebral areas most often produces nerve root impingement but also can cause compression of the spinal cord. Involvement of the cervical spine can develop within 2 years of the onset of RA. Severe, clinically significant spinal disease, however, tends to occur in long-standing active disease and usually is associated with extensive erosive disease of peripheral joints.[4–6] Treatment with disease-modifying antirheumatic drugs (DMARDs) and biological agents can prevent cervical spine disease but does not impact the progression of preexisting spinal instabilities.

Atlantoaxial Subluxation

The atlantoaxial (C1-C2) joint, which is the cervical spinal segment most commonly affected by RA, permits the widest range of motion of any spinal segment. As a consequence, the damaged atlantoaxial joints are exposed to stresses and strains that can predispose to anterior, posterior, lateral, rotational, or vertical subluxation.[7]

By far the most common abnormality is anterior subluxation of C1 on C2, which occurs when pannus develops in the synovial spaces surrounding the odontoid and weakens the transverse and alar ligaments. As a result, the anterior arch of C1, which normally is held tightly against the odontoid process of C2, migrates anteriorly, and the anterior atlantodental interval (the distance between the anterior arch of C1 and the odontoid) increases. Measurement of the anterior atlantodental interval is commonly used to detect atlantoaxial subluxation on plain radiographs with values greater than 3.0 mm and 4.5 mm, indicative of subluxation in adults and children, respectively. Impingement of the spinal cord, however, results from compromise of the spinal canal, which lies between the *posterior* arch of C1 and the odontoid. The spinal canal must accommodate the spinal cord (approximately 10 mm in diameter) as well as the dura mater and cerebrospinal fluid. The posterior atlantodental interval (the distance between the anterior aspect of the posterior arch of C1 and the posterior aspect of the odontoid) provides a measure of the diameter of spinal canal; the risk for cord compression increases when this interval is reduced to less than 14 mm.[8]

Other forms of atlantoaxial subluxation are less common. Lateral subluxation is due to asymmetric cartilage erosion; rotational subluxation occurs with transverse ligament damage. Posterior atlantoaxial subluxation develops when the dens, weakened by erosions and adjacent pannus, fractures, thereby allowing the anterior arch of C1 to migrate posteriorly. Posterior subluxation is uncommon but carries the greatest risk of severe neurologic compromise.[7] Vertical subluxation, which results from destruction of the lateral aspects of the atlantoaxial joint or the clivus (the basilar part of the occipital bone) or both, usually occurs in the context of atlantooccipital arthritis and is discussed as follows.

Symptoms and Signs of Atlantoaxial Subluxation

Atlantoaxial subluxation can be asymptomatic. Neck pain is a common but nonspecific symptom. A more specific symptom of atlantoaxial subluxation is severe, referred occipital pain due to compression of the exiting C2 nerve roots. There may be loss of cervical lordosis and resistance to passive motion of the spine. Lateral and rotational subluxation can result in head tilt. Most serious are symptoms pointing to impingement of the cervical spinal cord: weakness and sensory symptoms in the upper and lower extremities and sphincter dysfunction with retention and incontinence. In such cases, examination can demonstrate long tract signs consistent with a myelopathy: bilateral motor weakness with increased tone and spasticity, diffuse hyperreflexia, clonus, positive Hoffman signs, and extensor plantar reflexes. Weakness due myelopathy can easily be overlooked in the setting of destructive arthritis of large peripheral joints and the sarcopenia that can accompany long-standing, active RA. Once present, the symptoms and signs of spinal cord compression usually are progressive.

Vertical Subluxation due to Atlantooccipital Arthritis

The craniovertebral junction includes the occiput and the first 2 cervical vertebrae. Involvement of the atlantooccipital joint in RA usually occurs concomitantly with atlantoaxial inflammation and instability. Vertical subluxation at the craniovertebral junction (also known as cranial settling or basilar invagination) is a highly morbid complication of RA. Erosive damage to the atlantooccipital joint and the odontoid (sometimes leading to odontoid fracture) and weakening of the alar and apical ligaments permit upward movement of the odontoid. As the odontoid vertically penetrates the foramen magnum, serious complications arise from compression of cranial nerves, the vertebral arteries, the spinal cord, and the medulla. The clinical manifestations include compression neuropathies of the abducens, vagal, and hypoglossal cranial nerves; upper and lower extremity weakness and paresthesias, diffuse hyperreflexia, and extensor plantar reflexes due to upper cervical cord compression; cortical blindness, vertigo, nausea, tinnitus, and cerebellar dysfunction due to compromise of the posterior cerebral circulation; and apnea, drop-attacks, and sudden death due to medullary impingement.

Subaxial Cervical Spine Subluxation

Instability of the subaxial (C3-C7) joints manifests as horizontal subluxation of one vertebral body on another and stems from synovitis of the facet joints and damage to the intervertebral discs and interspinous ligaments. Subaxial subluxation can affect more than 1 level and can cause spinal cord compression or cervical nerve root compression or both.[7] Sensory symptoms due to nerve root impingement can result in pain and numbness that involves the shoulder (C5) or that radiates from the shoulder to the thumb (C6), to the index and long fingers (C7), or to the ring and little fingers (C8). Impingement of motor roots leads to loss of the biceps (C5/6) or triceps (C7) deep tendon reflexes or to weakness of the finger flexors (C8).

Imaging of the Cervical Spine in Rheumatoid Arthritis

Radiographic imaging plays a critical role in defining the extent and severity of cervical spine involvement in RA. Due to its ability to detect soft tissue and spinal cord abnormalities, MRI is the imaging modality of choice for patients with neurologic deficits. Computed tomography (CT) is the best means to evaluate boney changes and cervical instabilities before surgery, but has limited value in the evaluation for soft tissue changes or spinal cord compression. Plain radiography cannot detect spinal cord impingement, is relatively insensitive for the detection of erosions, and visualizes the craniocervical junction poorly. However, plain radiography is relatively inexpensive and is useful for screening of asymptomatic patients.

Plain radiographs of the cervical spine should include an anteroposterior view, lateral and flexion-extension views, and an open-mouth view of the odontoid (to assess lateral or rotatory atlantoaxial subluxation). Flexion views are most helpful for the detection of anterior atlantoaxial subluxation. The normal anterior atlantodental interval is less than 3 mm in adults and less than 4.5 mm in pediatric patients; intervals greater than these indicate anterior subluxation of C1 on C2 (**Figs. 1–3**).

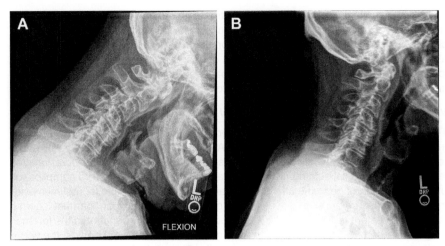

Fig. 1. Imaging of the cervical spine disease in a patient with long-standing, seropositive RA who developed refractory neck pain despite excellent control of his peripheral arthritis with anti–tumor necrosis factor therapy. (*A, B*) Plain lateral radiographs of the cervical spine in flexion (*A*) and extension (*B*) reveal significant anterior subluxation of C1 on C2 with an anterior atlantodental interval of 5 mm. There is extensive subaxial disease with subluxation of C3 on C4 and disc space narrowing, anterior osteophytosis, and facet joint disease of the lower cervical spine.

An anterior atlantodental interval greater than 8 mm suggests total rupture of the transverse and alar ligaments, but, as a general guide, the anterior atlantodental interval is an imperfect indicator of neurologic outcomes. The posterior atlantodental interval is better, with an increased risk for neurologic compromise observed when this index is less than 14 mm and poor outcomes seen with indices less than 10 mm.[8]

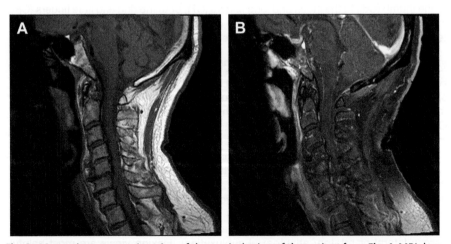

Fig. 2. Magnetic resonance imaging of the cervical spine of the patient from **Fig. 1**. MRI demonstrates marked erosive destruction of the dens without evidence of active articular inflammation or myelopathy. (*A, B*) There is severe foraminal narrowing and inflammatory facet joint arthritis of the lower cervical spine (*B*).

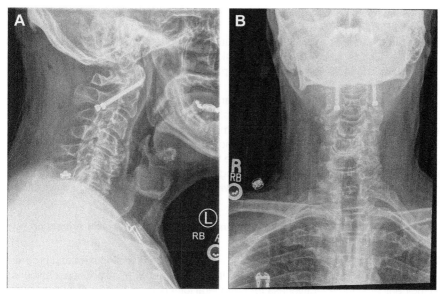

Fig. 3. Plain lateral *(A)* and anteroposterior *(B)* radiographs following successful posterior atlanotaxial fixation via transarticular screw placement for atlantoaxial subuxation due to rheumatoid arthritis.

Nonetheless, because plain radiographs do not visualize soft tissue abnormalities that can compromise the spinal canal, such as retro-odontoid pannus, spinal cord compression can occur in RA even when both the anterior and posterior atlantodental intervals are only minimally abnormal. Plain radiographs also have limitations when screening for vertical subluxation at the craniovertebral junction (cranial settling) due to the difficulties in delineating the structures at the base of the skull and the eroded tip of the odontoid process. This difficulty is reflected in the development of multiple criteria to diagnose cranial settling by plain radiography, not one of which has satisfactory sensitivity and specificity. As a consequence, MRI has supplanted plain radiography for assessment of vertical subluxation at the craniovertebral junction. Plain radiography does provide a reliable measure of spinal alignment. Subaxial subluxation is present with there is more than 2 mm of anterior displacement of one cervical vertebra on another and is considered severe when there is more than 4 mm of displacement. However, measurement of the sagittal diameter of the subaxial spinal canal, which normally ranges from 14 to 23 mm, better correlates with neurologic deficits.

MRI should be performed when there is suspicion of neurologic deficits attributable to RA involvement of the cervical spine or when screening plain radiography provides evidence of cervical instability. MRI is superior to other imaging modalities in its ability to assess spinal cord compression and nerve root impingement and to visualize the contribution of soft tissue inflammation, such as pannus formation, to spinal stenosis. MRI can be used to measure the cervicomedullary angle (the angle between the anterior spinal cord and the medulla) to detect vertical subluxation at the craniovertebral junction (less than 135° indicates cranial settling). MRI also can identify synovitis, pannus formation, and bone marrow edema pattern in juxta-articular bone before the development of structural abnormalities and thus is the most sensitive imaging modality for the detection of cervical spine involvement early in the course of RA.

CT scan is superior to MRI in the evaluation of bone anatomy but is limited in its ability to visualize spinal cord compression or soft tissue abnormalities, such as synovitis or pannus formation. It is particularly useful for planning surgical reconstruction.

MR angiography and CT angiography can define the anatomy of the vertebral artery circulation and are mandatory for preoperative evaluation before C1-2 fusion. Although the vertebral arteries have a simple vertical course in the subaxial spine, they make an acute but variable lateral bend within the body of C2. Preoperative delineation of the vascular anatomy can reduce to risk of inadvertent injury to the vertebral arteries during fixation surgery.[9] MR angiography and CT angiography also are useful in the assessment of the patient with RA with cervical spine instability and symptoms of vertebrobasilar insufficiency.

The Effect of Disease-Modifying Antirheumatic Drugs and Biological Agents on Cervical Spine Disease

Data on the effect of DMARDs and biological agents on the development and progression of cervical spine disease in RA are limited compared with the abundant evidence on their efficacy and effectiveness for peripheral joint damage. Nonetheless, one prospective study has established that the combination of methotrexate, sulfasalazine, and hydroxychloroquine administered for 2 years in early RA significantly reduces the prevalence of anterior atlantoaxial subluxation at 5 years of follow-up compared with monotherapy with sulfasalazine (3% vs 14%).[4] Retrospective cohort studies indicate that the development of de novo cervical spine lesions is uncommon among patients with RA patients treated with long-term biological agents but that the great majority of preexisting atlantoaxial and vertical subluxations progress despite treatment.[10] Thus, aggressive and effective medical management of RA with DMARDs and biologic agents appears to prevent the development of cervical spine disease, particularly when initiated early in the course of disease. Once spinal instabilities develop, however, these usually worsen despite medical management, perhaps because biomechanical forces are major drivers of deterioration once joint and ligamentous damage has occurred.[2,10]

Nonoperative Management

Nonoperative management of cervical instability with pain management, collars, and physical therapy may relieve discomfort but does not change the progression of cervical involvement in RA. These conservative measures, together with an aggressive medical management of RA disease activity and close monitoring, are appropriate initial therapy for patients with pain but no neurologic deficits. Because most patients with myelopathy experience neurologic deterioration in the absence of surgical intervention, conservative management is not appropriate if signs of myelopathy are present.

Operative Management

The universally accepted indications for surgery on the rheumatoid cervical spine are (1) neurologic deficits attributable to cervical spine disease and (2) pain that has failed nonoperative management. Because myelopathy is progressive and nonoperative interventions are ineffective, early aggressive surgical intervention is indicated for patients with neurologic deficits.[11] Patients with cervical or occipital pain but without neurologic signs and symptoms should receive a trial of conservative management.

If the pain proves to be intractable, surgical arthrodesis often is effective at ameliorating or eliminating pain.

A gray area is the patient who has significant cervical instability on imaging studies but who has no neurologic findings and minimal pain. The decision to intervene surgically is not trivial: not all such patients develop myelopathy; perioperative mortality in patients with RA ranges from 5% to 10%; and there is risk for morbidity from deep surgical infection, failure of arthrodesis due to osteopenic bone, and the development of pseudoarthrosis and subluxation below the site of fusion.[8,12] Because of the considerable morbidity and mortality of vertical subluxation, prophylactic surgical fusion usually is recommended if there is imaging evidence of vertical subluxation (eg, the cervicomedullary angle is <135° on MRI). In cases of asymptomatic atlantoaxial subluxation, some advocate for a period of observation if the posterior atlantodental interval is more than 14 mm, but favor operative intervention if MRI demonstrates a spinal canal that is less than 13 mm. Of note, dynamic MRI with flexion views can demonstrate significant narrowing of the spinal canal or even cord compression that is not seen when the neck is imaged in the neutral position.

A description of specific surgical approaches and methods is beyond the scope of this review. Because instability is the major problem of the rheumatoid cervical spine, all surgical approaches aim to achieve stability through the fusion of affected spinal elements (eg, atlantoaxial fixation for atlantoaxial subluxation, occipitospinal fusion for vertical subluxation). Outcomes are highly dependent on the extent of disease and neurologic deficits before surgery. For example, in a large, single-center series, Miyamoto and colleagues[13] reported the best long-term results for patients with isolated, reducible atlantoaxial subluxation and the poorest outcomes for patients with subaxial subluxations. Adjacent pseudoarthrosis and development of subaxial subluxations are serious complications of occipitospinal fusion for vertical subluxation; the incidence of these complications can be reduced by the use of longer fusions but at the cost of a higher rate of deep infection.

Special Considerations

Patients who have cervical spinal disease due to RA are especially susceptible to severe injury from falls, whiplash, hyperextension or hyperflexion, and endotracheal intubation. Because hyperextension during intubation can exacerbate cervical subluxation and precipitate compression of brainstem or spinal cord, even patients with asymptomatic RA who require intubation warrant preoperative cervical spine evaluation with radiography that must include flexion and extension views. Patients with RA with cervical disease require special care, including fiberoptic-guided intubation during general anesthesia.

RHEUMATOID MENINGITIS
Overview

Meningitis is a rare but serious manifestation of RA.[14,15] The meninges, which envelop the brain and spinal cord, consist of 3 membranes: the dura mater (outermost); the arachnoid mater; and the pia mater (the innermost membrane that adheres directly to brain and spinal cord). RA can affect each of these layers, causing pachymeningitis (inflammation of the dura mater), leptomeningitis (inflammation the arachnoid and pia mater), or a combination of pachymeningitis and leptomeningitis.[14,15] Rheumatoid meningitis can be patchy or diffuse and usually affects the meninges that surround the brain rather than the spinal cord.[14,15]

Rheumatoid meningitis is primarily, if not exclusively, a complication of seropositive RA. It occurs most often in long-standing disease and can develop in individuals whose articular disease is clinically quiescent.[14,15] Rheumatoid meningitis was rare before the introduction of effective therapies for RA, and it is not known whether aggressive and early disease-modifying therapy has further reduced its incidence, as appears to be the case with other forms of serious extra-articular disease.

Presentation and Diagnosis of Rheumatoid Meningitis

The presenting symptoms of rheumatoid meningitis are variable and likely are impacted by whether the meningitis is localized or diffuse, by its location, and by the meningeal layers affected (eg, pachymeningitis vs leptomeningitis). Headache is common, as are seizures, focal neurologic deficits, altered mental status, and cranial nerve abnormalities (due to compression from pachymeningitis).[14,15] As a general guide, rheumatoid meningitis should be considered whenever a patient with long-standing RA develops new neurologic findings that point to an intracranial process. Because rheumatoid meningitis is rare, however, imaging abnormalities usually first raise the possibility of this diagnosis.

Establishing the diagnosis of rheumatoid meningitis is difficult. Lumbar puncture typically reveals a modest lymphocytic pleocytosis and mildly elevated protein, but cerebrospinal fluid can be normal; the primary purpose of lumbar puncture is to help exclude infection.[15] The diagnosis is highly reliant on imaging, particularly MRI, and may require biopsy. Brain MRI shows thickening of the pachymeninges or leptomeninges or both with enhancement on extra-axial high-intensity fluid-attenuated inversion recovery or diffusion-weighted imaging.[16] Meningeal thickening and enhancement is usually focal but can be diffuse. Biopsy of lesions identified by MRI reveals a characteristic but nonspecific mononuclear cell infiltration of the affected meninges that often includes abundant plasma cells.[16] Rheumatoid nodules within the meninges are specific for rheumatoid meningitis. These are found in most autopsy cases but are seen less often in biopsy specimens. Granulomatous inflammation sometimes occurs; vasculitis is present in a minority of cases.[15,17]

Differential Diagnosis

The differential diagnosis of rheumatoid meningitis is broad. The initial presentation can mimic a wide range of neurologic processes (eg, strokes, subdural hematomas and other intracranial masses, indolent infections), but MRI findings serve to focus the differential diagnosis on infiltrative or chronic inflammatory diseases that can affect the meninges. These include chronic granulomatous infections with *Mycobacterium tuberculosis*, atypical mycobacteria, and fungi; meningovascular syphilis; neurosarcoid; antineutrophil cytoplasmic autoantibody–associated vasculitis, particularly granulomatosis with polyangitis; immunoglobulin (Ig)G4-related disease; lymphoma; and meningeal metastases. Clinical context and laboratory investigation can eliminate some of these alternative possibilities, but often biopsy is required.

Treatment of Rheumatoid Meningitis

There are no clinical trials to guide treatment for rheumatoid meningitis, which instead rests on the anecdotal experiences of case reports. Treatment modalities include glucocorticoids (usually initiated as intravenous pulses of methylprednisolone) alone or in combination with DMARDs, azathioprine, or cyclophosphamide.[15] Treatment attenuates but often does not completely resolve findings on MRI. Relapses can occur. One interesting report described a patient who had a high volume of CD20-expressing B lymphocytes on histopathology and who had a sustained remission following the administration of rituximab.[18]

COMPRESSION NEUROPATHIES

Compression neuropathies are the most common form of peripheral nervous system involvement in RA. Compression can result from synovitis, tenosynovitis, joint subluxation and other articular malalignments, and, rarely, rheumatoid nodules. The point prevalence of carpal tunnel syndrome in RA is approximately 10% in RA.[19] Studies of tarsal tunnel syndrome suggest a similar prevalence in RA but symptoms are typically mild and often overlooked.[20] Compressions of the ulnar nerve at the elbow or the wrist and of the posterior interosseous nerve at the elbow are uncommon to rare complications of RA.

Compression of the median nerve as it courses through the wrist (carpal tunnel syndrome) is common in RA but also is a prevalent condition in the general adult population. A recent meta-analysis concluded that RA confers an approximately twofold increased risk for carpal tunnel syndrome.[21] The median nerve provides sensory innervation for the palmar surface of the hand from the wrist to the thumb, index and long fingers, and for the dorsal surface of the index and long fingers; it innervates the thenar muscles and the lumbricals.[22,23] Classic early signs of carpal tunnel syndrome are paresthesias and numbness of the hand, especially at night or with activities that flex the wrist, such as typing or driving.[22,23] Symptoms also can radiate proximally along the volar aspect of the forearm. Tapping over the median nerve on the volar aspect of the wrist (Tinel sign) can elicit pain.[22] Flexing the wrist at 90° for 1 minute also may reproduce paresthesias and pain (Phalen sign). If there is progression to motor compromise, patients describe clumsiness as well as difficulty grasping objects and opening jars; on examination, there can be atrophy of the thenar eminence and diminished ability to oppose and abduct the thumb.[22]

Tarsal tunnel syndrome occurs when the posterior tibial nerve is compressed as it courses with the posterior tibial artery behind the medial malleolus and manifests as paresthesias and pain on the plantar aspect of foot.[23,24] Tapping over the tarsal tunnel (Tinel sign) elicits pain. Synovitis of the radiocapitellar joint of the elbow can compress the posterior interosseous nerve, a branch of the radial nerve, leading to aching pain in the extensor muscles of the forearm.[22,23] In its most severe form, entrapment of the posterior interosseous nerve can mimic ruptured extensor tendons with inability to extend at the metacarpals or the wrist.[22,23] The ulnar nerve can be compressed at the elbow (cubital tunnel syndrome) or wrist (Guyon canal syndrome).[22,23] The cubital tunnel syndrome presents as paresthesias of the small finger and the ulnar aspect of the ring finger; long-standing compression leads to weakness and atrophy of the intrinsic muscles of the hand.[22,23] Guyon canal syndrome causes paresthesias only on the palmar aspect of the ring and small fingers (the branch that provides sensory innervation to the dorsal ulnar aspect of the hand bifurcates off the ulnar nerve proximal to the Guyon canal).[22,23]

Most compressive neuropathies can be diagnosed clinically. Electromyography and nerve conduction studies can confirm the diagnosis and usually are required before surgery; false-negative results, however, are common with tarsal tunnel syndrome.[24] Imaging is usually not necessary except for unusual cases when there is suspicion for compressing tumors, cysts, or nodules; in these cases, MRI may point to the correct diagnosis. Ultrasound is a newer modality to assess compressive disease and is an attractive alternative due to cost, but results are user dependent.

Initial treatment modalities include rest, splinting, and local corticosteroid injections. Orthotics can be effective for tarsal tunnel syndrome orthotics.[22–24] Surgical decompression is indicated for refractory pain and sensory symptoms or if motor symptoms and signs are present.[22–24]

ISCHEMIC NEUROPATHY DUE TO RHEUMATOID VASCULITIS

A serious extra-articular manifestation of RA is a necrotizing arteritis that shares features with polyarteritis nodosa (PAN) and that, like PAN, can involve the vasa nervorum, leading to nerve ischemia.[25,26] This arteritis occurred in fewer than 1% of patients with RA when it was characterized in the 1960s and now is rare.[27] It should not be confused with the still common and more benign form of rheumatoid vasculitis that manifests primarily as nail-fold infracts.[26]

Rheumatoid arteritis usually is a complication of long-standing, erosive, rheumatoid factor–positive RA.[25,26] There is controversy whether male sex is a risk factor, as was once thought. Antecedent weight loss is common, but fever is not.[25] As is the case with PAN, peripheral nerve involvement is common in rheumatoid arteritis and manifests in several distinct clinical forms: mononeuritis, mononeuritis multiplex, multifocal sensory and motor neuropathy, and distal symmetric sensory neuropathy. Rheumatoid arteritis can affect other organ systems but, with the exception of skin, appears to do so less often that PAN.[25,26]

Laboratory abnormalities in rheumatoid arteritis include elevations of the erythrocyte sedimentation rate and other inflammatory markers.[25] Some patients have eosinophilia.[27] The prevalence of rheumatoid factor approaches 100%, and approximately 50% of patients have a positive test for antineutrophil cytoplasmic antibodies in a perinuclear pattern (but only 10% have antibodies to myeloperoxidase).[28] Hypocomplementemia may be present, often in the pattern of a low C4 with a normal C3.[25] Electrophysiologic studies can characterize the pattern of peripheral nerve abnormality, but definitive diagnosis requires biopsy.[25,26] Muscle should always be biopsied in addition to nerve (sural nerve or superficial peroneal nerve).[28]

As is the case with PAN, rheumatoid arteritis warrants aggressive therapy with high-dose glucocorticoids, and many patients require additional immunosuppression in the form of cyclophosphamide.[25,26] There is limited experience with the use of rituximab or other biological agents for this manifestation of RA.

REFERENCES

1. Joaquim AF, Appenzeller S. Cervical spine involvement in rheumatoid arthritis—a systematic review. Autoimmun Rev 2014;13:1195–202.
2. Neva MH, Häkkinen A, Mäkinen H, et al. High prevalence of asymptomatic cervical spine subluxation in patients with rheumatoid arthritis waiting for orthopaedic surgery. Ann Rheum Dis 2006;65:884–8.
3. Krauss WE, Bledsoe JM, Clarke MJ, et al. Rheumatoid arthritis of the craniovertebral junction. Neurosurgery 2010;66:83–95.
4. Kauppi M, Neva M, Laiho K. Rheumatoid atlantoaxial subluxation can be prevented by intensive use of traditional disease modifying antirheumatic drugs. J Rheumatol 2009;36:273–8.
5. Neva MH, Isomaki P, Hannonen P, et al. Early and extensive erosiveness in peripheral joints predicts atlantoaxial subluxations in patients with rheumatoid arthritis. Arthritis Rheum 2003;48:1808–13.

6. Elhai M, Wipff J, Bazeli R, et al. Radiological cervical spine involvement in young adults with polyarticular juvenile idiopathic arthritis. Rheumatology 2013;52: 267–75.
7. Bouchaud-Chabot A, Lioté F. Cervical spine involvement in rheumatoid arthritis, a review. Joint Bone Spine 2002;69:141–54.
8. Boden S, Dodge L, Bohlmann H, et al. Rheumatoid arthritis of the cervical spine. J Bone Joint Surg Am 1993;75:1282–97.
9. Neo M. Treatment of the upper cervical spine in rheumatoid arthritis patients. Mod Rheumatol 2008;18:327–35.
10. Kaito T, Ohshima S, Fujiwara H, et al. Predictors for the progression of cervical lesion in rheumatoid arthritis under the treatment of biological agents. Spine 2013;38:2258–63.
11. Ostrowski RA, Takagishi T, Robinson J. Rheumatoid arthritis, spondyloarthropathies, and relapsing polychondritis. Handb Clin Neurol 2014;119:449–61.
12. Hohl J, Grabowski G, Donaldson W. Cervical deformity in rheumatoid arthritis. Semin Spinal Surg 2011;23:181–7.
13. Miyamoto H, Sumi M, Uno K. Outcome of surgery for the rheumatoid spine at one institute over three decades. Spine J 2013;13:1477–84.
14. Bathon JM, Moreland LW, DiBartolomeo AG. Inflammatory central nervous system involvement in rheumatoid arthritis. Semin Arthritis Rheum 1989;18:258–66.
15. Kato T, Hoshi K, Sekijima Y, et al. Rheumatoid meningitis: an autopsy report and review of the literature. Clin Rheumatol 2003;22:475–80.
16. Jones SE, Belsley NA, McLoud TC, et al. Rheumatoid meningitis: radiologic and pathologic correlation. Am J Roentgenol 2006;186:1181–3.
17. Yeaney GA, Denby EL, Jahromi BS, et al. Rheumatoid-associated meningitis and vasculopathy. Neurology 2015;84:1717–8.
18. Schmid L, Müller M, Treumann T, et al. Induction of complete and sustained remission of rheumatoid pachymeningitis by rituximab. Arthritis Rheum 2009; 60:1632–4.
19. Agarwal V, Singh R, Wiclaf, et al. A clinical, electrophysiological, and pathological study of neuropathy in rheumatoid arthritis. Clin Rheumatol 2008;27:841–4.
20. McGuigan L, Burke D, Fleming A. Tarsal tunnel syndrome and peripheral neuropathy in rheumatoid disease. Ann Rheum Dis 1983;42:128–31.
21. Shiri R. Arthritis as a risk factor for carpal tunnel syndrome: a meta-analysis. Scand J Rheumatol 2016;45:339–46.
22. Johnston JC, Deune EG. Approach to the patient with hand, wrist, or elbow pain. In: Imboden JB, Hellmann DB, Stone JH, editors. Current diagnosis and treatment rheumatology. 3rd edition. New York: McGraw Hill; 2013. p. 41–56.
23. Muramatsu K, Tanaka H, Taguchi T. Peripheral neuropathies of the forearm and hand in rheumatoid arthritis: diagnosis and options for treatment. Rheumatol Int 2008;28:951–7.
24. Ahmad M, Tsang K, Mackennery PJ, et al. Tarsal tunnel syndrome: a literature review. Foot Ankle Surg 2012;18:149–52.
25. Puechal X, Said G, Hilliquin P, et al. Peripheral neuropathy with necrotizing vasculitis in rheumatoid arthritis. Arthritis Rheum 1995;38:1618–29.
26. Genta MS, Genta RM, Gabay C. Systemic rheumatoid vasculitis: a review. Semin Arthritis Rheum 2006;36:88–98.
27. Schneider HA, Yonker RA, Katz P, et al. Rheumatoid vasculitis: experience with 13 patients and review of the literature. Semin Arthritis Rheum 1985;14:280–6.
28. Voskuyl AE, Hazes JMW, Zwinderman AH, et al. Diagnostic strategy for the assessment of rheumatoid vasculitis. Ann Rheum Dis 2003;62:407–13.

Central Nervous System Disease in Antineutrophil Cytoplasmic Antibodies–Associated Vasculitis

Jonathan Graf, MD

KEYWORDS

- Antineutrophil cytoplasmic antibodies (ANCA) • Granulomatosis with polyangiitis
- Microscopic polyangiitis
- Eosinophilic granulomatosis with polyangitiis (Churg-Strauss syndrome)
- Chronic hypertrophic pachymeningitis • Pituitary pseudoadenoma

KEY POINTS

- Central nervous system disease is an uncommon manifestation of granulomatosis with polyangiitis, is rare in microscopic polyangiitis, and does not occur in eosinophilic granulomatosis with polyangiitis.
- The 3 most important central nervous system manifestations of granulomatosis with polyangiitis are chronic hypertrophic pachymeningitis, pituitary disease, and cerebral vasculitis.
- Treatment of ANCA-associared CNS vasculitis often involves combination immunosuppressive regimens that include high dose corticosteroids and cytoxic agents or rituximab.

OVERVIEW

The antineutrophil cytoplasmic antibodies (ANCA)-associated diseases, granulomatosis with polyangiitis (GPA), microscopic polyangiitis (MPA), and eosinophilic granulomatosis with polyangiitis (EGPA), are primary systemic vasculitic diseases. GPA is an idiopathic granulomatous necrotizing small-vessel vasculitis associated with ANCA primarily directed against proteinase 3 (PR3). Its most common clinical manifestations are granulomatous vasculitis with sinonasal inflammation and necrosis, cavitary pulmonary masses and diffuse alveolar hemorrhage, and a crescentic, pauci-immune glomerulonephritis.[1] MPA is a systemic vasculitis of small- to medium-sized vessels

Dr J. Graf has no disclosures and no conflicts of interest.
Division of Rheumatology, University of California, Zuckerberg San Francisco General Hospital, San Francisco, 1001 Potrero Avenue, Box 0868, San Francisco, CA 94143, USA
E-mail address: Jonathan.Graf@ucsf.edu

Rheum Dis Clin N Am 43 (2017) 573–578
http://dx.doi.org/10.1016/j.rdc.2017.06.006
0889-857X/17/© 2017 Elsevier Inc. All rights reserved.

rheumatic.theclinics.com

that is associated with antibodies directed against the target antigen myeloperoxidase (MPO). It usually manifests as glomerulonephritis and diffuse alveolar hemorrhage.[2] Nevertheless, both GPA and MPA are systemic disorders that can affect organ systems other than the airways and kidneys, including the central nervous system (CNS). In contrast to GPA and MPA, CNS involvement in EGPA or in PAN is very rare, if it occurs at all.

CNS involvement in GPA is widely reported and affects between 7% and 11% of GPA patients, a figure that is even higher if cranial neuropathies are also included as manifestations.[3,4] Generally, when GPA affects the CNS, it tends to involve 3 primary structures: the pituitary gland, the meninges, and the cerebral vasculature.[3,4] Although the cause of GPA remains unknown, its predilection for these areas is thought to be related to 3 distinct pathogenic mechanisms.[3] First, GPA is unique among the ANCA-associated diseases in its ability to cause granulomatous inflammation capable of invading neighboring structures. Because inflammation in GPA commonly originates in the sinonasal structures, GPA can invade the orbit, optic nerve, chiasma, cranial nerves, meninges, and pituitary gland. Second, granulomatous inflammation can occur remotely in the CNS and involve the cerebrum, meninges, cranial nerves, and parietal bone. Finally, GPA is a systemic disease, and vasculitis of small and medium arteries can occur in the CNS, including cerebral and spinal vessels, much as it can occur elsewhere in the body.[3]

PITUITARY INVOLVEMENT

Pituitary involvement is an uncommon but widely recognized complication of GPA, affecting 1.3% of GPA patients in one large longitudinal cohort.[5] Another retrospective series of 819 patients with GPA diagnosed between 1963 and 2014 reported pituitary involvement in 1.1%.[6] The median age of diagnosis of pituitary disease in these 2 studies was 48 and 50, respectively, with men and women being evenly affected in both cohorts.[5,6] Three different pathogenic mechanisms of pituitary disease have been suggested, including in situ development of granulomatous inflammation in the gland itself and vasculitis of the pituitary vessels.[5] However, the most widely accepted mechanism implicates granulomatous invasion of the pituitary from neighboring sinus cavities, a notion suggested by the observation that 16 of 17 patients in the 2 largest series of GPA-associated pituitary disease also had concomitant upper airway involvement.[5,6] Other disease manifestations of GPA were also common, with approximately one-third of patients with pituitary disease having glomerulonephritis, and others having dermatitis, arthritis, and central or peripheral nervous system involvement.[5–7]

GPA-associated hypophysitis can lead to partial or global pituitary dysfunction.[8] Both the anterior and the posterior pituitary can be affected and lead in some cases to panhypopituitarism.[5] Patients initially complain of nonspecific symptoms, including headache, generalized weakness, and fatigue, which can delay recognition of this condition. With more pronounced pituitary involvement, clinical symptoms often will reflect specific endocrinopathies. Diabetes insipidus, a sign of posterior pituitary involvement, is the most commonly reported manifestation of GPA-related pituitary dysfunction, with patients complaining of polyuria and polydipsia with elevated serum but depressed urine osmolality.[5,6,9] Secondary hypogonadism, reflecting involvement of the anterior pituitary, is also prominent and can cause menstrual dysregulation, decreased libido, loss of muscle mass, erectile dysfunction, and diminished testicular size.[5,6] Secondary hypothyroidism from diminished Thyroid Stimulating hormone production, adrenal insufficiency from reduced production of adrenal corticotropic hormone, and growth hormone deficiency have all been reported as well. Hyperprolactinemia and galactorrhea can develop when granulomatous inflammation compresses the pituitary stalk, and a characteristic pattern of visual loss can occur if pituitary enlargement compresses the optic chiasm.

The differential diagnosis of GPA-associated pituitary disease includes other infectious and inflammatory granulomatous diseases, such as tuberculosis, sarcoidosis, Crohn disease, giant cell arteritis, and idiopathic giant cell granulomatosis, as well as a lymphocytic predominant form of primary hypophysitis.[8] ANCA has been shown to be positive in most patients, including 7 of 8 patients who demonstrated antibodies to PR3 as reported in one series and 3 of 3 in another.[5,8] Complete pituitary function should be assessed in all individuals with GPA suspected of having pituitary involvement. MRI evaluation is abnormal in up to 90% of patients[7] and usually demonstrates enlargement of the pituitary gland or a sellar mass with peripheral enhancement and central cystic changes suggestive of necrosis.[5,8] Other findings include compression of the pituitary stalk and infundibular thickening and enhancement. Histologic diagnosis is not necessary when a patient has other organ involvement and a clinical and serologic picture strongly suggestive of GPA. However, when MRI is obtained to evaluate headache or sinus disease, it can reveal an unexpected, isolated pituitary abnormality in the absence of other clinical manifestations of GPA. In cases where pituitary involvement is the only disease manifestation, where other diagnoses are suspected, or where response to treatment is not as expected, it may be necessary to obtain tissue for histopathologic evaluation.[5]

Pituitary involvement in GPA is most commonly treated with classical induction regimens for systemic vasculitis, including high-dose corticosteroids and cyclophosphamide.[5,6,8] Alternative immunosuppressive agents have also been used and include rituximab, azathioprine, mycophenolate mofetil, methotrexate, and infliximab.[5,7,8] However, although clinical remission has been reported in up to 69% of patients receiving one of these immunosuppressive regimens, relapses appear to be lower in those patients who are initially treated with cyclophosphamide (11%) compared with other agents (>50%).[6] Cyclophosphamide appears to be especially preferable to rituximab, the latter of which is reported to be more effective for vasculitis-associated disease than for control of granulomatous inflammation, the component of GPA most often implicated in pituitary disease.[6] Despite clinical and radiologic evidence of remission or improvement in GPA, patients are often left with long-term pituitary deficits, sometimes requiring life-long replacement therapy. One case series of 3 patients reported persistent pituitary dysfunction in every patient after achievement of remission from GPA.[8] Another reported resolution of normal pituitary function in only 17% of patients who otherwise achieved remission.[7,10] One reason may be that granulomatous inflammation induces early, substantive, and potentially irreversible damage to the pituitary cells.[6]

MENINGEAL INVOLVEMENT

Meningeal involvement is a widely recognized but rare manifestation of ANCA-associated vasculitis, most commonly associated with GPA. The pachymeninges are more frequently involved than the leptomeninges, and although inflammatory lesions can occur throughout the dura, GPA more often infiltrates the intracranial rather than the spinal dura matter.[9] Granulomatous inflammation causes thickening of the dura and can present clinically with a range of symptoms that include headache, cranial neuropathies, cerebellar ataxia, seizures, myelopathy, and neuroophthalmologic complications.[9,11,12] When it occurs, chronic hypertrophic pachymeningitis (CHP) is more often an initial presenting manifestation of GPA rather than a later complication of disease, with up to 60% of CHP presenting at disease onset.[9,12]

It remains unclear whether ANCA-associated CHP is a single entity or heterogeneous group of diseases. ANCA with specificity for either PR3 or MPO has been observed in different patients with CHP. Whether all ANCA-associated CHP is related to GPA regardless of ANCA specificity or whether anti-MPO–positive patients have MPA or an entirely different disease is uncertain, but there is growing evidence to suggest that serologic specificity in CHP correlates with both clinical features and overall prognosis. This is especially true for anti-PR3–positive CHP patients who are more likely to have systemic disease that includes pulmonary and renal vasculitis.[11] Conversely, anti-MPO–positive patients are more likely to be older women with a CNS-limited form of the disease that has less severe neurologic involvement and lower levels of inflammatory markers such as C-reactive protein.[11]

There are also many similarities as well between CHP patients who are anti-PR3 or anti-MPO positive. The frequency of chronic sinusitis, otitis media, mastoiditis, and retroorbital pseudotumor has been found to be generally similar in both PR3- and MPO-positive patients, and the MRI appearance of both groups has demonstrated similar patterns of dural thickening, with the PR3-positive patients more likely to have parenchymal and leptomeningeal involvement.[11] Histopathologically, both anti-PR3– and anti-MPO–positive disease demonstrate dural thickening and fibrosis, with some biopsies also showing necrotizing granulomatous inflammation with vasculitis within the thickened dura.[11,12]

Treatment of ANCA-associated CHP is based on regimens that consist of cyclophosphamide or other immunosuppressives plus high-dose corticosteroid therapy, because combination therapy with cyclophosphamide demonstrates greater efficacy with fewer relapses than corticosteroid-only regimens.[11] Rituximab has also been shown to benefit patients with active and even refractory CHP in other published series.[12–15] Annual relapse rates for anti-PR3–associated disease are approximately double that of anti-MPO–positive disease, the same ratio that is seen in patients with anti-PR3– and anti-MPO–associated glomerulonephritis.[11,16] Thus, anti-PR3– and anti-MPO–positive CHP may be 2 distinct entities, and, although their clinical, radiologic, and histologic appearance in the CNS may be similar, the severity of disease and response to treatment may be very different. Anti-PR3–associated disease appears to resemble systemic GPA with pachymeningeal involvement, whereas anti-MPO–positive CHP is more likely to be limited to the CNS and relapse less frequently, analogous to patients with anti-MPO–positive renal-limited vasculitis.[11]

CEREBRAL VASCULITIS

As is the case with other systemic vasculitides, both GPA and MPA can cause inflammation within the vasculature of the CNS.[3,17,18] Vascular inflammation can result in ischemic or hemorrhagic damage to the brain parenchyma and spinal cord with resultant focal or generalized neurologic deficits.[19] This primarily vascular phenotype is in contrast to the predominantly (although not exclusively) granulomatous phenotype described in cases of pituitary and pachymeningeal disease.[19] Ischemic complications are most common and can cause transient ischemic attack or stroke with motor deficits, ischemic myelopathy, encephalopathy, cognitive impairment and dementia, mood disorders, seizures, and cortical blindness.[18–25] When present, hemorrhage can occur within the cerebral cortex or the subarachnoid space.[26]

Diagnosis of cerebral vasculitis can be challenging because the differential diagnosis is broad and includes infectious and neoplastic diseases. Furthermore, although MRI is sensitive for detecting ischemic lesions within the CNS, it is relatively nonspecific and can show both large cerebral infarctions and extensive white matter lesions, consistent with small-vessel ischemic disease.[19] Computed tomography, MRI, and conventional angiography only occasionally demonstrate aneurismal or stenotic lesions or both, because the size of the involved vessels is frequently below the level of resolution of these imaging techniques.[3,4] Lumbar puncture and cerebral spinal fluid analysis may demonstrate nonspecific abnormalities such as elevated protein and pleocytosis but help to rule out infectious, neoplastic, or other disease in the differential diagnosis.[19] Therefore, the diagnosis is often clinically based and relies on recognition of extracranial symptoms and serologies consistent with a diagnosis of ANCA-associated vasculitis in the appropriate clinical context. In extreme cases where the diagnosis remains uncertain, cerebral biopsy can help confirm the diagnosis.[3]

Treatment of ANCA-associated CNS vasculitis is similar to that used for other severe organ-threatening manifestations of GPA and MPA. Combination regimens consisting of high-dose corticosteroids plus intravenous or oral cyclophosphamide or rituximab are mainstays of induction therapy.[3,4,19,24,25] In extreme cases, plasma exchange has also been used.[24] Long-term maintenance therapy with azathioprine or other immunosuppressive agents is recommended after achieving remission during the induction phase of treatment.[19]

REFERENCES

1. Stone JH. Granulomatosis with polyangiitis (wegener granulomatosis). Chapter 32. In: Imboden JB, Hellmann DB, Stone JH, editors. Current diagnosis & treatment: rheumatology. New York: The McGraw-Hill Companies; 2013. Available at: accessmedicine.mhmedical.com/content.aspx?aid=57273174. Accessed June 16, 2017.

2. Duvuru G, Stone JH. Microscopic polyangiitis. Chapter 33. In: Imboden JB, Hellmann DB, Stone JH, editors. Current diagnosis & treatment: rheumatology. New York: The McGraw-Hill Companies; 2013. Available at: accessmedicine. mhmedical.com/content.aspx?aid=57273266. Accessed June 16, 2017.

3. Seror R, Mahr A, Ramanoelina J, et al. Central nervous system involvement in Wegener granulomatosis. Medicine (Baltimore) 2006;85(1):54–65.

4. Ghinoi A, Zuccoli G, Pipitone N, et al. Anti-neutrophil cytoplasmic antibody (ANCA)-associated vasculitis involving the central nervous system: case report and review of the literature. Clin Exp Rheumatol 2010;28(5):759–66.

5. Kapoor E, Cartin-Ceba R, Specks U, et al. Pituitary dysfunction in granulomatosis with polyangiitis: the Mayo Clinic experience. J Clin Endocrinol Metab 2014; 99(11):3988–94.

6. De Parisot A, Puéchal X, Langrand C, et al. Pituitary involvement in granulomatosis with polyangiitis: report of 9 patients and review of the literature. Medicine (Baltimore) 2015;94(16):e748.

7. Yong TY, Li JYZ, Amato L, et al. Pituitary involvement in Wegener's granulomatosis. Pituitary 2008;11(1):77–84.

8. Esposito D, Trimpou P, Giugliano D, et al. Pituitary dysfunction in granulomatosis with polyangiitis. Pituitary 2017;20(5):594–601.

9. Holle JU, Gross WL. Neurological involvement in Wegener's granulomatosis. Curr Opin Rheumatol 2011;23(1):7–11.

10. Slabu H, Arnason T. Pituitary granulomatosis with polyangiitis. BMJ Case Rep 2013;2013 [pii:bcr2013008656].
11. Yokoseki A, Saji E, Arakawa M, et al. Hypertrophic pachymeningitis: significance of myeloperoxidase anti-neutrophil cytoplasmic antibody. Brain 2014;137(Pt 2): 520–36.
12. Shimojima Y, Kishida D, Hineno A, et al. Hypertrophic pachymeningitis is a characteristic manifestation of granulomatosis with polyangiitis: a retrospective study of anti-neutrophil cytoplasmic antibody-associated vasculitis. Int J Rheum Dis 2017;20(4):489–96.
13. Sharma A, Kumar S, Wanchu A, et al. Successful treatment of hypertrophic pachymeningitis in refractory Wegener's granulomatosis with rituximab. Clin Rheumatol 2010;29(1):107–10.
14. Just SA, Knudsen JB, Nielsen MK, et al. Wegener's granulomatosis presenting with pachymeningitis: clinical and imaging remission by rituximab. ISRN Rheumatol 2011;2011:608942.
15. Jang Y, Lee ST, Jung KH, et al. Rituximab treatment for idiopathic hypertrophic pachymeningitis. J Clin Neurol 2017;13(2):155–61.
16. Lionaki S, Blyth ER, Hogan SL, et al. Classification of antineutrophil cytoplasmic autoantibody vasculitides: the role of antineutrophil cytoplasmic autoantibody specificity for myeloperoxidase or proteinase 3 in disease recognition and prognosis. Arthritis Rheum 2012;64(10):3452–62.
17. Fauci AS, Haynes BF, Katz P, et al. Wegener's granulomatosis: prospective clinical and therapeutic experience with 85 patients for 21 years. Ann Intern Med 1983;98(1):76–85.
18. Shuai ZW, Lv YF, Zhang MM, et al. Clinical analysis of patients with myeloperoxidase antineutrophil cytoplasmic antibody-associated vasculitis. Genet Mol Res 2015;14(2):5296–303.
19. De Luna G, Terrier B, Kaminsky P, et al. Central nervous system involvement of granulomatosis with polyangiitis: clinical-radiological presentation distinguishes different outcomes. Rheumatology (Oxford) 2015;54(3):424–32.
20. Reinhold-Keller E, de Groot K, Holl-Ulrich K, et al. Severe CNS manifestations as the clinical hallmark in generalized Wegener's granulomatosis consistently negative for antineutrophil cytoplasmic antibodies (ANCA). A report of 3 cases and a review of the literature. Clin Exp Rheumatol 2001;19(5):541–9.
21. Hoffman GS, Kerr GS, Leavitt RY, et al. Wegener granulomatosis: an analysis of 158 patients. Ann Intern Med 1992;116(6):488–98.
22. Payton CD, Jones JM. Cortical blindness complicating Wegener's granulomatosis. Br Med J (Clin Res Ed) 1985;290(6469):676.
23. Mattioli F, Capra R, Rovaris M, et al. Frequency and patterns of subclinical cognitive impairment in patients with ANCA-associated small vessel vasculitides. J Neurol Sci 2002;195(2):161–6.
24. Isoda K, Nuri K, Shoda T, et al. Microscopic polyangiitis complicated with cerebral infarction and hemorrhage: a case report and review of literature. Nihon Rinsho Meneki Gakkai Kaishi 2010;33(2):111–5.
25. Zhang W, Zhou G, Shi Q, et al. Clinical analysis of nervous system involvement in ANCA-associated systemic vasculitides. Clin Exp Rheumatol 2009;27(1 Suppl 52):S65–9.
26. Cruz DN, Segal AS. A patient with Wegener's granulomatosis presenting with a subarachnoid hemorrhage: case report and review of CNS disease associated with Wegener's granulomatosis. Am J Nephrol 1997;17(2):181–6.

Neuromyelitis Optica

Sarah L. Patterson, MD, Sarah E. Goglin, MD*

KEYWORDS

- Neuromyelitis optica • Longitudinally extensive transverse myelitis • Optic neuritis
- Area postrema syndrome • Aquaporin-4

KEY POINTS

- Neuromyelitis optica spectrum disorders (NMOSD) are rare inflammatory diseases of the central nervous system caused by astrocyte injury and secondary demyelination.
- It manifests clinically as acute, recurrent attacks of optic neuritis complicated by vision loss, longitudinally extensive transverse myelitis, and/or area postrema syndrome (intractable hiccups or nausea/vomiting).
- Aquaporin-4 autoantibodies (AQP4-IgG) are pathogenic, and detection in the serum confers moderate sensitivity and high specificity for the disease.
- Current treatment involves aggressive immunosuppression with pulse-dose steroids during acute attacks and long-term immunosuppression for attack prevention.

INTRODUCTION

Neuromyelitis optica (NMO) and neuromyelitis optica spectrum disorders (NMOSDs) are rare antibody-mediated disorders of the central nervous system (CNS) with a predilection for the spinal cord and optic nerves.[1] The hallmark manifestations are recurrent longitudinally extensive transverse myelitis and optic neuritis (ON). NMOSD was previously thought to be a variant of multiple sclerosis (MS), but the identification of aquaporin 4–immunoglobulin G (AQP4-IgG; also known as NMO-IgG), a serologic antibody against AQP4, has led to an appreciation of these diseases as distinct entities. Whereas older diagnostic criteria defined NMO and NMOSD separately based on clinical criteria, the newest diagnostic criteria define a single diagnosis under the term NMOSD.

EPIDEMIOLOGY

Cases of NMO have been reported across all major ethnic groups, with a reported prevalence that ranges broadly across studies between 0.5 and 10 per 100,000.[2–5]

Drs S. Patterson and S.E. Goglin have no financial disclosures and no conflicts of interest.
Division of Rheumatology, Department of Medicine, University of California, San Francisco, 400 Parnassus Avenue, San Francisco, CA 94143, USA
* Corresponding author. University of California, San Francisco, Box 0633, San Francisco, CA 94143.
E-mail address: Sarah.Goglin@ucsf.edu

Rheum Dis Clin N Am 43 (2017) 579–591
http://dx.doi.org/10.1016/j.rdc.2017.06.007
0889-857X/17/© 2017 Elsevier Inc. All rights reserved.

rheumatic.theclinics.com

Similar to other autoimmune disorders, there is a strong female predilection. In the case of the more common recurrent form of the disease, which represents 80% to 90% of cases, women are overrepresented with a ratio of 5 to 10:1.[6] The median age of onset is 39,[7] which differs from most patients with MS for whom the first manifestation is younger, typically between ages 20 and 40 years.[5,6,8]

The frequency of NMO/NMOSD is roughly the same worldwide, but cohort studies demonstrate a slightly higher proportion of AQP4-antibody–positive patients among Asian individuals with idiopathic demyelinating CNS diseases compared with whites.[1] Additionally, US cohort studies suggest higher prevalence among self-identified blacks.[4] This observation was supported by a population-based study that compared incidence and prevalence across 2 different counties. The prevalence in Olmsted County, Minnesota, a primarily Caucasian community, is 3.9 per 100,000 compared with 10 per 100,000 in Martinique, an island in the eastern Caribbean Sea where Afro-Caribbean ethnicity predominates.[5] The ethnicity-specific prevalence in these 2 counties was similar and 2.4 times higher among blacks relative to whites.

PATHOPHYSIOLOGY

In contrast to MS, NMO is more accurately considered an astrocytopathy as opposed to a primary demyelinating disease. Studies in animals and humans suggest a pathophysiologic model in which AQP4-IgG autoantibodies produced in the periphery enter the CNS where they bind astrocyte foot processes, inducing complement-mediated cell damage, granulocyte infiltration, and astrocyte death.[9–13] Astrocyte death results in secondary oligodendrocyte death, demyelination, and ultimately neuronal cell death. Mature NMO lesions demonstrate pan-necrosis with widespread infiltration of macrophages surrounded by AQP4-positive reactive astrocytes.[10]

Several studies in vitro and in vivo have demonstrated the importance of AQP4-IgG (also known as NMO-IgG) in the etiopathogenesis of NMO.[9–14] Aquaporin 4 is a water-selective channel that is predominately expressed in the CNS where it functions by facilitating bidirectional water flow across cell membranes in response to osmotic gradients.[10] Investigators have reproduced NMO lesions by injecting immunoglobulin from patients seropositive for NMO along with human complement into mice brains.[12] Seven days after injection, the animal brains develop key histologic features of NMO, including extensive inflammatory cell infiltrate, perivascular deposition of activated complement, loss of aquaporin-4 expression, demyelination, and neuronal cell death.

The pathogenicity and clinical relevance of AQP4-IgG has been confirmed in human studies. Patients with high serum antibody titers demonstrate higher disease activity and longer spinal cord damage on MRI during exacerbations.[13,14] Patients with high titers are also at increased risk for complete blindness and large cerebral lesions on MRI.[13] In a longitudinal study of 8 seropositive patients, serum antibody levels declined significantly after treatment with immunosuppressive agents, such as rituximab, azathioprine, or cyclophosphamide.[14]

The absence of autoantibody generation intrathecally in patients with NMO suggests that AQP4-IgG is produced in the periphery and enters the CNS secondarily.[15,16] Researchers have identified a subpopulation of interleukin (IL)-6–dependent B cells (CD27+ CD38+ CD180−) that are increased in the peripheral blood of patients with NMO and produce most of AQP4-IgG.[17] These B cells are morphologically and phenotypically identical to plasmablasts, expand during NMO relapse, and increase AQP4-IgG production in response to IL-6 signaling. Furthermore, blockade of IL-6 by anti-IL-6 receptor antibody reduces plasmablast survival in vitro, therefore raising interest in IL-6 inhibition as a therapy for this disease.[17]

There are many aspects of the pathogenesis of NMO that remain unknown, including the following: (1) mechanism for loss of tolerance and autoantibody (AQP4-IgG) formation; (2) pathogenesis of seronegative NMO/NMOSD; and (3) mechanisms by which AQP4-IgG breach the blood-brain barrier.

CLINICAL PRESENTATION

The classic clinical manifestation of NMO is recurrent acute attacks of transverse myelitis and/or unilateral or bilateral ON with incomplete recovery between attacks.[6,7,18–20] Following the discovery of AQP4-IgG, there has been increased awareness of additional potential clinical manifestations, including brainstem and cerebral syndromes, leading to revised diagnostic criteria published by the International Panel for NMO Diagnosis (IPND) in 2015 (see "diagnostic criteria" section later in this article).[21] Attacks are characterized by neurologic deficits that develop over days with variable resolution during subsequent months, leading to progressive disability.[20,22] Most patients (80%–90%) suffer from recurrent disease, and relapses often occur early at unpredictable intervals. In a review of 71 patients with NMO evaluated at the Mayo Clinic, the second relapse occurred within 1 year in 60% and within 3 years in 90% of patients with relapsing disease.[20]

Transverse Myelitis

The term "transverse myelitis" (TM) represents a heterogeneous group of inflammatory disorders characterized by bilateral sensorimotor and autonomic spinal cord dysfunction, spinal cord inflammation by cerebrospinal fluid (CSF) analysis or MRI, and exclusion of compressive, postradiation, and vascular causes.[23–26] TM can result from a variety of underlying infectious, demyelinating, and autoimmune conditions. Other autoimmune causes of TM, which may coexist with NMOSD, include systemic lupus erythematosus, Sjogren syndrome, antiphospholipid syndrome, and neurosarcoidosis. TM in the setting of NMOSD is often severe, resulting in paraparesis or quadriparesis, bladder dysfunction, and sensory loss caudal to the level of the cord lesion.[6]

Imaging by MRI most commonly demonstrates "longitudinally extensive transverse myelitis" (LETM), lesions extending over 3 or more spinal cord segments, involving the cervical or thoracic cord (**Fig. 1**). Lesions show a central cord predominance with most of the lesion residing within the central gray matter, and acute lesions tend to encompass most of the cross-sectional area with associated swelling and gadolinium enhancement.[6,27,28]

Optic Neuritis

ON, inflammation of the optic nerve, presents with vision loss and eye pain exacerbated by eye movement. Compared with MS, ON in NMO is more severe and more likely to present with simultaneous bilateral or rapidly sequential eye involvement.[6] During an acute attack, MRI may show increased signal on fat-suppressed T2-weighted sequences (**Fig. 2**) or T1 gadolinium enhancement in the optic nerve or optic chiasm.[6,21] The lesions are typically long, extending more than half the distance from orbit to optic chiasm, and involve the posterior aspect of the nerve or the chiasm. In patients with acute ON, 84% show increased signal intensity on T2-weighted short-tau inversion recovery scans of the optic nerve,[29] and 94% demonstrate gadolinium enhancement on T1-weighted spin-echo sequences.[30]

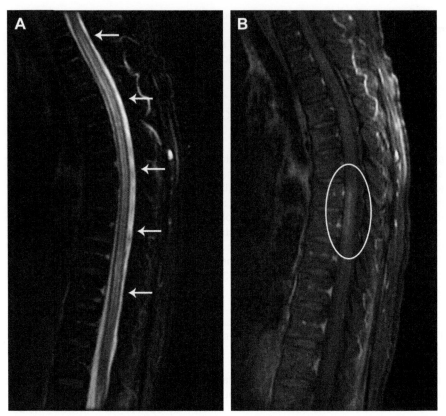

Fig. 1. Spinal cord MRI from patient with acute LETM in the setting of AQP4-IgG–positive NMOSD. Panel A shows abnormal increased signal (*arrows*) on sagittal T2-weighted sequence extending throughout thoracic cord and lower cervical cord. Panel B demonstrates abnormal gadolinium enhancement (*circle*) in lower thoracic cord on sagittal T1-weighted sequence.

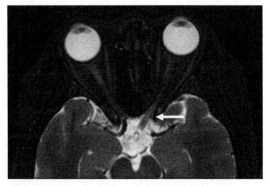

Fig. 2. Optic nerve MRI from a patient with NMOSD and acute ON. T2-weighted MRI in the axial plane shows increased signal in the posterior aspect of the left optic nerve.

Brainstem Syndromes

The area postrema syndrome results from involvement of the medulla and presents clinically with intractable hiccups and/or nausea and vomiting. It can manifest radiographically with lesions involving the dorsal medulla (especially the area postrema), but only a small percentage of patients with NMO/NMOSD and acute vomiting or hiccups have corresponding MRI lesions detectable by conventional imaging techniques.[21,31] In an international multicenter study of 258 patients with NMO, brainstem signs were common, affecting 31% of the cohort, and occurred most commonly as part of the initial attack (54%) or early in the course of the disease.[31] The most common signs were vomiting (33%), hiccups (22%), oculomotor dysfunction (20%), and pruritus (12%). Other reported deficits from brainstem involvement include hearing loss, facial palsy, vertigo, vestibular ataxia, and trigeminal neuralgia.

DIAGNOSTIC EVALUATION

The initial diagnostic evaluation should include serologic testing for AQP4-IgG, neuroimaging of the brain and spine, CSF analysis, and ophthalmologic evaluation.

Serum Aquaporin 4–Immunoglobulin G Testing

Testing for serum AQP4-IgG is an important part of the diagnostic evaluation. It demonstrates moderate sensitivity and high specificity for the disease, although precise test characteristics vary depending on the specific assay that is used. The initial assay based on indirect immunofluorescence method had a reported sensitivity of 58% to 75% and specificity of 85% to 99%, whereas cell-based assays have both higher sensitivity (74%–83%) and specificity (100%).[5,32–34] A small proportion of seronegative patients who meet criteria for NMOSD are subsequently found to be AQP4-IgG positive, and it is therefore recommended that they be retested at the time of recurrent attacks. Additionally, because titers increase during relapse and decline following treatment in some individuals, retesting should be considered before initiating treatment with immunosuppressing and antibody-targeted therapies.[21] However, there are no data to support regular testing of antibody levels in patients with confirmed disease, as investigators have not identified a threshold at which relapse can be predicted.[14,35]

Cerebrospinal Fluid

CSF studies should include cell count, cytology, protein, albumin CSF–serum ratio, immunoglobulin (IgG, IgA, IgM) CSF–serum ratios, and oligoclonal bands (OCBs).[36] CSF can be helpful in distinguishing NMOSD from MS, as there are well-documented differences. For example, NMOSD is more likely to cause pleocytosis (incidence approximately 35% in NMOSD), particularly the presence of neutrophils or eosinophils, and less associated with the presence of oligoclonal bands.[21] Patients with NMOSD also demonstrate an increase in CSF IL-6, which is not observed in patients with MS.[1] CSF AQP4-IgG is rarely positive in patients with negative serum antibody testing and therefore unlikely to add diagnostic utility.

Ophthalmologic Examination

On examination, patients with ON will demonstrate decreased color vision or "red desaturation" (red objects look orange or gray from the affected eye). They also may have bland optic disc swelling on fundus examination, and if there is unilateral involvement, an afferent pupillary defect.

Neuroimaging

Neuroimaging is an important aspect of the diagnostic evaluation, particularly in patients with clinical features consistent with NMOSD who are AQP4-IgG negative. Patients should undergo MRI with and without gadolinium enhancement of the brain and spine, as well as dedicated optic nerve MRI in cases concerning for ON. Imaging findings associated with the most common clinical syndromes are described in the "clinical presentation" section.

DIAGNOSTIC CRITERIA

The diagnostic criteria were revised by the IPND and published in 2015.[21] In contrast to previously published criteria, the newer criteria use nomenclature that defines the unifying term NMOSDs, which is stratified by serologic testing into seropositive and seronegative disease. The definition for seronegative disease requires that patients meet more stringent clinical criteria with additional neuroimaging findings. The newer criteria recognize clinical manifestations of the disease beyond optic nerve and spinal cord involvement and define 6 "core clinical characteristics." These core characteristics and the specific diagnostic criteria for seropositive and seronegative disease are outlined in **Box 1**.

DIFFERENTIAL DIAGNOSIS

The hallmark feature of NMO is LETM, for which the differential diagnosis includes infectious, autoimmune, demyelinating, and paraneoplastic syndromes. Important diseases to consider within each of these categories are summarized in **Box 2**. Of note, as many as 29% of patients ultimately diagnosed with NMO/NMOSD are initially misdiagnosed with MS,[4] and it is critical to distinguish between these diseases, as certain treatments used in MS, such as interferon-β, can worsen disease activity in NMO. Laboratory features that are helpful in distinguishing NMO from MS include anti-AQP4 antibody positivity (present in 70%–90% of patients with NMO/NMOSD vs negative in MS) and absence of CSF OCBs (CSF OCBs present in 15% of patients with NMO/NMOSD vs 80% of MS). Neuroimaging is also often critical for distinguishing between NMO and MS, as the cord lesions of MS tend to be located peripherally and typically involve short segments spanning less than 1 vertebral length,[37] as opposed to the longitudinally extensive cord lesions typical of NMO/NMOSD.

TREATMENT: ACUTE ATTACK

Both initial and recurrent episodes should be treated with high-dose steroids. The standard regimen is methylprednisolone 1 g intravenous daily for 3 to 5 days, followed by an oral steroid taper. Oral steroids are generally continued until sufficient time has elapsed for the chosen steroid-sparing immunosuppressive agent (see the following section on "attack prevention") to take full effect. Therapeutic plasma exchange is recommended as part of acute therapy in cases refractory to high-dose steroids and also should be considered in episodes involving spinal cord demyelination.[6,38,39]

TREATMENT: ATTACK PREVENTION

Once the diagnosis of NMOSD is confirmed, long-term immunosuppression should be initiated early. The goals of therapy in this context are to delay time to relapse, reduce the severity of future attacks, and minimize permanent disability. Given the rarity of the disease, there are no randomized controlled trials to guide treatment decisions.

Box 1
Diagnostic criteria for neuromyelitis optica spectrum disorders (NMOSDs)

Core clinical characteristics

- Optic neuritis

- Acute myelitis

- Area postrema syndrome (episodes of otherwise unexplained hiccups or nausea and vomiting)

- Acute brainstem syndrome

- Symptomatic narcolepsy or acute diencephalic clinical syndrome with NMOSD-typical diencephalic MRI lesions

- Symptomatic cerebral syndrome with NMOSD-typical brain lesions

Diagnostic criteria for NMOSD with Aquaporin 4–immunoglobulin G (AQP4-IgG)

1. At least 1 core clinical characteristic

2. Positive test for AQP4-IgG using best available detection method

3. Exclusion of alternative diagnoses

Diagnostic criteria for NMOSD without AQP4-IgG or antibody status unknown

1. At least 2 core clinical characteristics meeting all of the following characteristics:
    a. At least 1 core clinical characteristic must be optic neuritis, acute myelitis with longitudinally extensive transverse myelitis (LETM), or area postrema syndrome
    b. Dissemination in space (2 or more different core clinical characteristics)
    c. Fulfillment of additional MRI requirements
        i. Acute optic neuritis: brain MRI shows normal findings or nonspecific white matter lesions; OR optic nerve MRI demonstrates T2-hyperintense lesion or T1-weighted gadolinium enhancing lesion extending over at least half the optic nerve length or involving optic chiasm
        ii. Acute myelitis: spine MRI lesion extending over at least 3 contiguous segments (LETM)
        iii. Area postrema syndrome: associated dorsal medulla lesions
        iv. Acute brainstem syndrome: associated periependymal brainstem lesions

2. Negative test for AQP4-IgG, or testing unavailable

3. Exclusion of alternative diagnoses

Adapted from Wingerchuk DM, Banwell B, Bennett JL, et al. International consensus diagnostic criteria for neuromyelitis optica spectrum disorders. Neurology 2015;85(2):177–89.

However, observational studies show improved outcomes with several immunosuppressive agents, including rituximab, mycophenolate mofetil (MMF), azathioprine (AZA), and mitaxantrone.[36,40–42]

Rituximab

Several open-label studies have shown a reduction in relapse rate and disability following treatment with rituximab, and most experts consider it first-line therapy for attack prevention.[43–46] In a review of open-label studies of patients with NMOSD treated with rituximab, a mean 64% of patients were relapse free at follow-up, which ranged from 12 to 67 months.[44] In a long-term study of 30 patients with NMOSD treated with repeated rituximab, 87% maintained a marked reduction in relapse rate, 93% had improvement or stability in disability over 5 years of follow-up, and there was no increased safety risk with long-term B-cell depletion.[45] The adverse events of

---

Box 2
Differential diagnosis of transverse myelitis

Demyelinating

- Multiple sclerosis
- Neuromyelitis optica
- Idiopathic transverse myelitis
- Acute disseminated encephalomyelitis

Infectious

- Bacterial
  ○ Syphilis, *Mycobacterium tuberculosis*, Lyme disease
- Viral
  ○ Herpes simplex virus type-2, varicella-zoster virus, cytomegalovirus, Epstein-Barr virus, coxsackie virus, enterovirus, hepatitis A and C
- Parasitic
  ○ Neurocysticercosis, *Schistosoma*, *Gnathostoma* angiostrongylosis
- Fungal
  ○ *Actinomyces*, *Coccidioides immitis*, *Aspergillus*, *Blastomyces dermatitidis*

Paraneoplastic

- Antiamphiphysin (breast carcinoma)
- Anti-CRMP-5 (small cell lung cancer)

Autoimmune/Inflammatory

- Systemic lupus erythematosus
- Sjogren syndrome
- Antiphospholipid syndrome
- Neurosarcoidosis
- Behcet disease
- Mixed connective tissue disease

Data from Refs.[24,61,62]

---

rituximab in the setting of NMOSD are similar to those observed in other conditions, such as rheumatoid arthritis, including infusion reactions and infections.[44]

Treatment with rituximab is initiated with either 2 infusions of 1 g spaced 2 weeks apart or 4 weekly 375-mg/m^2 body surface area administrations. A variety of regimens for maintenance therapy have been tried, including redosing every 6 to 9 months, redosing when the CD19 population exceeds 0.1%, or with the therapeutic target of ≤0.05% circulating peripheral memory B cells (CD27+ cells in peripheral blood mononuclear cells).[44,45] Although data suggest an increased risk of relapse with repopulation of CD27+ memory cells,[45] there are no data from randomized controlled trials to support the superiority of one maintenance approach over the others.

Other Immunosuppressive Agents

MMF and AZA have been shown in observational studies to have moderate efficacy and acceptable safety for relapse prevention. In a French study of 67 patients with NMOSD treated with MMF, 51% had relapse while on treatment; however, 60%

continued treatment, 83% had stabilization or improvement in disability, and the median annualized relapse rate decreased from 1 pretreatment to 0 posttreatment.[40] Similarly, a study on the efficacy of AZA in 99 patients with NMO/NMOSD demonstrated reduced relapse rate, stabilization or improvement in disability, and improved visual acuity after treatment compared with pretreatment measures.[42] Although there are case series to support the use of mitoxantrone for relapse prevention,[47,48] its use is limited by its unfavorable side-effect profile (cardiotoxicity, therapy-related acute leukemia) and restricted duration of therapy. Cyclophosphamide and methotrexate also have been used to treat this disease, but efficacy data are insufficient to support their use as first-line agents.[36]

EMERGING THERAPIES
Eculizumab

Most AQP4-IgGs are from the IgG1 subclass, which avidly activates complement, and the membrane attack complex of the complement cascade leads to astrocyte damage that is central to the pathogenesis of NMOSD. Due to the understanding of the importance of complement activation in the pathogenesis of NMOSD, there is interest in targeted treatments against components of the complement cascade. Eculizumab is a humanized monoclonal antibody against complement protein C5. Through its neutralization of C5, it inhibits its cleavage to C5a and C5b and thus prevents generation of the proinflammatory and cell-activating C5a peptide, the terminal membrane attack complex C5b-9, and the soluble C5b-9 inflammatory component. It is currently approved for the treatment of paroxysmal nocturnal hemoglobinuria and atypical hemolytic uremic syndrome. It is currently under investigation for treatment of NMOSD. The results of an open-label pilot study were published in *Lancet Neurology* in 2013.[49] Fourteen patients with AQP4-IgG–seropositive NMOSD with at least 2 attacks in the preceding 6 months or at least 3 attacks in the preceding 12 months were enrolled. Of the 14 patients, 6 had failed previous treatment and 5 had not been treated with relapse prevention treatments before inclusion in the study. Subjects received 600 mg intravenous eculizumab weekly for 4 weeks, 900 mg in the fifth week, and then 900 mg every 2 weeks for 48 weeks. The primary endpoints were efficacy, which was measured by number of attacks, and safety. After 12 months of treatment, 12 patients were relapse free; 2 had had possible attacks. One patient had meningococcal sepsis and sterile meningitis 2 months after the first eculizumab infusion, but no other drug-related serious adverse events occurred. Eight attacks in 5 patients were reported within 12 months of eculizumab withdrawal. Further study of eculizumab in randomized controlled trials is warranted based on these results.

Tocilizumab

IL-6 is also postulated to play a role in the pathogenesis of NMOSD. Increased IL-6 levels have been detected in the serum and CSF of patients with NMOSD, especially during relapses. IL-6 also promotes AQP4-IgG production and secretion from plasmablasts. Tocilizumab, a humanized monoclonal antibody against the IL-6 receptor approved for the treatment of rheumatoid arthritis and giant cell arteritis, has shown early promise in small, uncontrolled studies of patients with NMOSD. Several case reports and a prospective pilot study demonstrated that tocilizumab administered for 12 to 24 months reduced clinical and MRI disease activity of NMO.[50–55] These results were confirmed in a retrospective study evaluating longer-term treatment with tocilizumab (up to 51 months) in 8 patients with severe relapsing disease that had been refractory to other therapies, including rituximab.[56]

Novel Therapeutics Targeting Aquaporin 4–Immunoglobulin G and Aquaporin 4

Novel therapeutics that block AQP4-IgG binding to AQP4 or inactivation of AQP4-Ig are an area of active investigation. "Aquaporumab" is a nonpathogenic monoclonal antibody generated from recombinant monoclonal AQP4-IgG that binds to AQP4. It competitively displaces pathogenic AQP4-IgGs in NMO patient sera, preventing complement-mediated and cell-mediated cytotoxicity. Additionally, it has been shown to reduce NMO lesions in spinal cord slice cultures in mice receiving intracerebral AQP4-IgG and complement.[57]

PROGNOSIS

The prognosis of NMOSD is generally poor, with high levels of associated disability. In a German study of 871 NMOSD attacks among 185 patients, only 22% showed full recovery and 6% showed no recovery at all.[38] Factors independently associated with a more favorable outcome included absence of myelitis (eg, isolated ON), younger age at disease onset, complete remission following the first attack, and lower attack frequency during the first year.[38,58] Roughly half of patients have severe visual defects or motor impairment within 5 years of disease onset.[58,59] The most common cause of disease-related mortality is neurogenic respiratory failure, and reported mortality rates in cohort studies range from 23% to 50% in cohort studies.[58–60] These outcomes are expected to improve as advances in NMOSD pathogenesis lead to improvements in treatment including more targeted therapies.

REFERENCES

1. Uzawa A, Mori M, Kuwabara S. Neuromyelitis optica: concept, immunology and treatment. J Clin Neurosci 2014;21(1):12–21.
2. Cabrera-Gomez JA, Kurtzke JF, González-Quevedo A, et al. An epidemiological study of neuromyelitis optica in Cuba. J Neurol 2009;256(1):35–44.
3. Asgari N, Lillevang ST, Skejoe HP, et al. A population-based study of neuromyelitis optica in Caucasians. Neurology 2011;76(18):1589–95.
4. Mealy MA, Wingerchuk DM, Greenberg BM, et al. Epidemiology of neuromyelitis optica in the United States: a multicenter analysis. Arch Neurol 2012;69(9):1176–80.
5. Flanagan EP, Cabre P, Weinshenker BG, et al. Epidemiology of aquaporin-4 autoimmunity and neuromyelitis optica spectrum. Ann Neurol 2016;79:775–83.
6. Sellner J, Boggild M, Clanet M, et al. EFNS guidelines on diagnosis and management of neuromyelitis optica. Eur J Neurol 2010;17(8):1019–32.
7. Wingerchuk DM, Lennon VA, Lucchinetti CF, et al. The spectrum of neuromyelitis optica. Lancet Neurol 2007;6(9):805–15.
8. Confavreux C, Vukusic S. The clinical epidemiology of multiple sclerosis. Neuroimaging Clin N Am 2008;18(4):589–622, ix–x.
9. Hinson SR, Pittock SJ, Lucchinetti CF, et al. Pathogenic potential of IgG binding to water channel extracellular domain in neuromyelitis optica. Neurology 2007;69(24):2221–31.
10. Papadopoulos MC, Verkman AS. Aquaporin 4 and neuromyelitis optica. Lancet Neurol 2012;11(6):535–44.
11. Ratelade J, Zhang H, Saadoun S, et al. Neuromyelitis optica IgG and natural killer cells produce NMO lesions in mice without myelin loss. Acta Neuropathol 2012;123(6):861–72.

12. Saadoun S, Waters P, Bell BA, et al. Intra-cerebral injection of neuromyelitis optica immunoglobulin G and human complement produces neuromyelitis optica lesions in mice. Brain 2010;133(Pt 2):349–61.
13. Takahashi T, Fujihara K, Nakashima I, et al. Anti-aquaporin-4 antibody is involved in the pathogenesis of NMO: a study on antibody titre. Brain 2007;130(Pt 5): 1235–43.
14. Jarius S, Aboul-Enein F, Waters P, et al. Antibody to aquaporin-4 in the long-term course of neuromyelitis optica. Brain 2008;131(Pt 11):3072–80.
15. Jarius S, Franciotta D, Paul F, et al. Cerebrospinal fluid antibodies to aquaporin-4 in neuromyelitis optica and related disorders: frequency, origin, and diagnostic relevance. J Neuroinflammation 2010;7:52.
16. Jarius S, Paul F, Franciotta D, et al. Cerebrospinal fluid findings in aquaporin-4 antibody positive neuromyelitis optica: results from 211 lumbar punctures. J Neurol Sci 2011;306(1–2):82–90.
17. Chihara N, Aranami T, Sato W, et al. Interleukin 6 signaling promotes anti-aquaporin 4 autoantibody production from plasmablasts in neuromyelitis optica. Proc Natl Acad Sci U S A 2011;108(9):3701–6.
18. Kim SH, Kim W, Li XF, et al. Clinical spectrum of CNS aquaporin-4 autoimmunity. Neurology 2012;78(15):1179–85.
19. Ghezzi A, Bergamaschi R, Martinelli V, et al. Clinical characteristics, course and prognosis of relapsing Devic's Neuromyelitis Optica. J Neurol 2004;251(1):47–52.
20. Wingerchuk DM, Hogancamp WF, O'Brien PC, et al. The clinical course of neuromyelitis optica (Devic's syndrome). Neurology 1999;53(5):1107–14.
21. Wingerchuk DM, Banwell B, Bennett JL, et al. International consensus diagnostic criteria for neuromyelitis optica spectrum disorders. Neurology 2015;85(2): 177–89.
22. Drori T, Chapman J. Diagnosis and classification of neuromyelitis optica (Devic's syndrome). Autoimmun Rev 2014;13(4–5):531–3.
23. Beh SC, Greenberg BM, Frohman T, et al. Transverse myelitis. Neurol Clin 2013; 31(1):79–138.
24. West TW, Hess C, Cree BA. Acute transverse myelitis: demyelinating, inflammatory, and infectious myelopathies. Semin Neurol 2012;32(2):97–113.
25. West TW. Transverse myelitis–a review of the presentation, diagnosis, and initial management. Discov Med 2013;16(88):167–77.
26. Transverse Myelitis Consortium Working Group. Proposed diagnostic criteria and nosology of acute transverse myelitis. Neurology 2002;59(4):499–505.
27. Nakamura M, Miyazawa I, Fujihara K, et al. Preferential spinal central gray matter involvement in neuromyelitis optica. An MRI study. J Neurol 2008;255(2):163–70.
28. Krampla W, Aboul-Enein F, Jecel J, et al. Spinal cord lesions in patients with neuromyelitis optica: a retrospective long-term MRI follow-up study. Eur Radiol 2009; 19(10):2535–43.
29. Johnson G, Miller DH, MacManus D, et al. STIR sequences in NMR imaging of the optic nerve. Neuroradiology 1987;29(3):238–45.
30. Kupersmith MJ, Alban T, Zeiffer B, et al. Contrast-enhanced MRI in acute optic neuritis: relationship to visual performance. Brain 2002;125(Pt 4):812–22.
31. Kremer L, Mealy M, Jacob A, et al. Brainstem manifestations in neuromyelitis optica: a multicenter study of 258 patients. Mult Scler 2014;20(7):843–7.
32. Lennon VA, Wingerchuk DM, Kryzer TJ, et al. A serum autoantibody marker of neuromyelitis optica: distinction from multiple sclerosis. Lancet 2004;364(9451): 2106–12.

33. Marignier R, Bernard-Valnet R, Giraudon P, et al. Aquaporin-4 antibody-negative neuromyelitis optica: distinct assay sensitivity-dependent entity. Neurology 2013; 80(24):2194–200.
34. Fryer JP, Lennon VA, Pittock SJ, et al. AQP4 autoantibody assay performance in clinical laboratory service. Neurol Neuroimmunol Neuroinflamm 2014;1(1):e11.
35. Pellkofer HL, Krumbholz M, Berthele A, et al. Long-term follow-up of patients with neuromyelitis optica after repeated therapy with rituximab. Neurology 2011; 76(15):1310–5.
36. Trebst C, Jarius S, Berthele A, et al. Update on the diagnosis and treatment of neuromyelitis optica: recommendations of the Neuromyelitis Optica Study Group (NEMOS). J Neurol 2014;261(1):1–16.
37. McDonald WI, Compston A, Edan G, et al. Recommended diagnostic criteria for multiple sclerosis: guidelines from the international panel on the diagnosis of multiple sclerosis. Ann Neurol 2001;50(1):121–7.
38. Kleiter I, Gahlen A, Borisow N, et al. Neuromyelitis optica: evaluation of 871 attacks and 1,153 treatment courses. Ann Neurol 2016;79(2):206–16.
39. Watanabe S, Nakashima I, Misu T, et al. Therapeutic efficacy of plasma exchange in NMO-IgG-positive patients with neuromyelitis optica. Mult Scler 2007;13(1): 128–32.
40. Montcuquet A, Collongues N, Papeix C, et al. Effectiveness of mycophenolate mofetil as first-line therapy in AQP4-IgG, MOG-IgG, and seronegative neuromyelitis optica spectrum disorders. Mult Scler 2016. 1352458516678474.
41. Kimbrough DJ, Fujihara K, Jacob A, et al. Treatment of neuromyelitis optica: review and recommendations. Mult Scler Relat Disord 2012;1(4):180–7.
42. Collongues N, de Seze J. Current and future treatment approaches for neuromyelitis optica. Ther Adv Neurol Disord 2011;4(2):111–21.
43. Collongues N, Brassat D, Maillart E, et al. Efficacy of rituximab in refractory neuromyelitis optica. Mult Scler 2016;22(7):955–9.
44. Collongues N, de Seze J. An update on the evidence for the efficacy and safety of rituximab in the management of neuromyelitis optica. Ther Adv Neurol Disord 2016;9(3):180–8.
45. Kim SH, Huh SY, Lee SJ, et al. A 5-year follow-up of rituximab treatment in patients with neuromyelitis optica spectrum disorder. JAMA Neurol 2013;70(9): 1110–7.
46. Kim SH, Kim W, Li XF, et al. Repeated treatment with rituximab based on the assessment of peripheral circulating memory B cells in patients with relapsing neuromyelitis optica over 2 years. Arch Neurol 2011;68(11):1412–20.
47. Kim SH, Kim W, Park MS, et al. Efficacy and safety of mitoxantrone in patients with highly relapsing neuromyelitis optica. Arch Neurol 2011;68(4):473–9.
48. Cabre P, Olindo S, Marignier R, et al. Efficacy of mitoxantrone in neuromyelitis optica spectrum: clinical and neuroradiological study. J Neurol Neurosurg Psychiatry 2013;84(5):511–6.
49. Pittock SJ, Lennon VA, McKeon A, et al. Eculizumab in AQP4-IgG-positive relapsing neuromyelitis optica spectrum disorders: an open-label pilot study. Lancet Neurol 2013;12(6):554–62.
50. Araki M, Aranami T, Matsuoka T, et al. Clinical improvement in a patient with neuromyelitis optica following therapy with the anti-IL-6 receptor monoclonal antibody tocilizumab. Mod Rheumatol 2013;23(4):827–31.
51. Araki M, Matsuoka T, Miyamoto K, et al. Efficacy of the anti-IL-6 receptor antibody tocilizumab in neuromyelitis optica: a pilot study. Neurology 2014;82(15):1302–6.

52. Ayzenberg I, Kleiter I, Schröder A, et al. Interleukin 6 receptor blockade in patients with neuromyelitis optica nonresponsive to anti-CD20 therapy. JAMA Neurol 2013;70(3):394–7.
53. Kieseier BC, Stüve O, Dehmel T, et al. Disease amelioration with tocilizumab in a treatment-resistant patient with neuromyelitis optica: implication for cellular immune responses. JAMA Neurol 2013;70(3):390–3.
54. Lauenstein AS, Stettner M, Kieseier BC, et al. Treating neuromyelitis optica with the interleukin-6 receptor antagonist tocilizumab. BMJ Case Rep 2014;2014 [pii:bcr2013202939].
55. Rose-John S, Gold R. Devic disease: translational medicine at work. Neurology 2014;82(15):1294–5.
56. Ringelstein M, Ayzenberg I, Harmel J, et al. Long-term therapy with interleukin 6 receptor blockade in highly active neuromyelitis optica spectrum disorder. JAMA Neurol 2015;72(7):756–63.
57. Tradtrantip L, Zhang H, Saadoun S, et al. Anti-aquaporin-4 monoclonal antibody blocker therapy for neuromyelitis optica. Ann Neurol 2012;71(3):314–22.
58. Cabre P, González-Quevedo A, Bonnan M, et al. Relapsing neuromyelitis optica: long term history and clinical predictors of death. J Neurol Neurosurg Psychiatry 2009;80(10):1162–4.
59. Wingerchuk DM, Weinshenker BG. Neuromyelitis optica: clinical predictors of a relapsing course and survival. Neurology 2003;60(5):848–53.
60. Papais-Alvarenga RM, Carellos SC, Alvarenga MP, et al. Clinical course of optic neuritis in patients with relapsing neuromyelitis optica. Arch Ophthalmol 2008; 126(1):12–6.
61. Cree BA. Acute inflammatory myelopathies. Handb Clin Neurol 2014;122:613–67.
62. Kitley JL, Leite MI, George JS, et al. The differential diagnosis of longitudinally extensive transverse myelitis. Mult Scler 2012;18(3):271–85.

Neurosarcoidosis

Patompong Ungprasert, MD[a,b,*], Eric L. Matteson, MD, MPH[a,c]

KEYWORDS

- Sarcoidosis • Neurosarcoidosis • Clinical manifestation • Imaging study
- Treatment • Outcome

KEY POINTS

- Neurosarcoidosis occurs in 3% to 10% of patients with sarcoidosis.
- Any part of the nervous system can be affected with cranial neuropathy and meningeal involvement being the most common manifestations.
- Glucocorticoids are the main therapy, although immunosuppressive agents are also often required because of the high rate of relapse.

INTRODUCTION

Sarcoidosis is a chronic granulomatous disease of unknown cause characterized by the presence of noncaseating granuloma.[1,2] Incidence of sarcoidosis differs considerably among ethnic groups and sexes, ranging from less than 1 new case per 100,000 per year among Japanese men to more than 70 new cases per 100,000 among African American women.[3–5] Sarcoidosis can virtually affect any organ including the nervous system with the reported prevalence of neurologic involvement between 3% and 10% of patients.[3,5–8] However, the true prevalence of neurosarcoidosis could be much higher as post-mortem studies report that only half of patients with neurosarcoidosis were recognized antemortem.[9,10]

CLINICAL FEATURES

Any part of the nervous system can be affected by sarcoidosis, and multiple lesions are often noted.[11–13] The frequency of each neurologic manifestation is summarized in **Table 1**. Neurologic abnormalities are one of the first clinical manifestations that

Disclosure Statement: The authors have no financial or nonfinancial potential conflicts of interest to declare.
[a] Division of Rheumatology, Department of Internal Medicine, Mayo Clinic College of Medicine and Science, 200 First Avenue Southwest, Rochester, MN 55905, USA; [b] Division of Rheumatology, Department of Medicine, Faculty of Medicine Siriraj Hospital, Mahidol University, 2 Prannok Road, Bangkok 10700, Thailand; [c] Division of Epidemiology, Department of Health Science Research, Mayo Clinic College of Medicine and Science, 200 First Avenue Southwest, Rochester, MN 55905, USA
* Corresponding author. Division of Rheumatology, Mayo Clinic, 200 First Avenue Southwest, Rochester, MN 55905.
E-mail addresses: P.Ungprasert@gmail.com; Ungprasert.Patompong@mayo.edu

Rheum Dis Clin N Am 43 (2017) 593–606
http://dx.doi.org/10.1016/j.rdc.2017.06.008
0889-857X/17/© 2017 Elsevier Inc. All rights reserved.

Table 1
Frequency of each neurologic manifestation among patients with neurosarcoidosis	
Neurologic Manifestation	**Frequency, %**
Facial nerve neuropathy	11–25
Optic neuritis	7–35
Vestibulocochlear nerve involvement	3–17
Meningitis	10–20
Intraparenchymal brain lesions on imaging studies	Up to 50
Seizure	15
Depression	60
Neuroendocrinologic dysfunction	2–8
Spinal cord involvement	5–20
Peripheral neuropathy	2–86

lead to the diagnosis of sarcoidosis in 70% to 80% of patients with neurosarcoidosis.[13–15] Isolated neurosarcoidosis is uncommon, because more than 90% of patients also have sarcoidosis in other organs, especially the lungs and mediastinal lymph nodes.[5,11–13] One study found that more than 80% of patients with an initial diagnosis of isolated neurosarcoidosis eventually developed extraneurologic sarcoidosis over the course of more than 6.6 years of follow-up.[14]

Cranial Neuropathy

Cranial neuropathy is the most common manifestation of neurosarcoidosis. Involvement of all cranial nerves has been reported, with cranial nerve II, VII, and VIII being the most frequently affected.[16] An older cohort suggested that facial nerve palsy accounted for two-thirds of neurosarcoidosis.[15] More recent studies report that facial nerve palsy occurs in 11% to 25% of cases.[12–14,16,17] About one-third of facial nerve palsies are bilateral and could be either concurrent or sequential.[12,15,16]

It was formerly thought that facial nerve palsy is a consequence of sarcoidosis-associated inflammation of the parotid gland as classically described as Heerfordt syndrome.[18] However, more recent studies have failed to demonstrate a relationship between the 2 conditions. One study reported that only 20% of patients with facial nerve palsy had associated parotitis,[15] whereas another study reported no facial nerve palsy in 7 patients with parotitis due to sarcoidosis.[19] Epineural inflammation, perineural inflammation, and external compression by granulomatous mass/inflammation in leptomeninges are now more commonly accepted as the cause of cranial neuropathies, including facial nerve palsy.[16] The prognosis of cranial nerve involvement is generally good with complete recovery in more than 85% of cases.[13,15,20]

Optic neuritis accounts for 7% to 35% neurosarcoidosis cases.[13–17] Bilateral involvement is slightly more common than unilateral disease.[14,16,17] Typical presentations include subacute visual loss, retrobulbar pain, and papilledema on examination.[11] Outcome of optic neuritis is quite unfavorable. In one series with average duration of follow-up of 5 years, 30% of patients had visual acuity of 20/200 or worse at last follow-up.[17] Another series revealed a significant improvement of visual acuity in only 5 out of 18 patients during 18 months of follow-up.[21]

Involvement of vestibulocochlear nerve resulting in intermittent or persistent sensorineural hearing loss and vestibular dysfunction is seen in 3% to 17% of patients with neurosarcoidosis.[14,16,20,21] It is thought to be a consequence of granulomatous meningitis.[22]

Meningeal Involvement

Meningitis accounts for 10% to 20% of cases of neurosarcoidosis, although the frequency of subclinical leptomeningeal involvement detected on imaging studies is much higher.[14,15,21] Patients typically present with subacute to chronic onset of headache, constitutional symptoms, and signs of meningeal irritation.[23–25] Cerebrospinal fluid (CSF) analysis usually reveals monocyte pleocytosis, elevated protein level, and negative microbial cultures.[14,17,26] Hypoglycorrhachia is uncommon, detected in less than 15% of cases.[14,17] Noncaseating granuloma is found in about two-thirds of meningeal biopsies. Prognosis is generally favorable because the disease tends to respond well to treatment with glucocorticoids even though recurrence is common, and complications, such as seizure and communicating hydrocephalus, may occur.[11,15,23,24]

Brain Parenchymal Disease

Patients with brain parenchymal disease may present with seizure, headache, or cognitive/behavioral problems.[23] Seizures may be focal or generalized and are generally associated with intracranial mass, encephalopathy, vasculopathy, or hydrocephalus.[27] Seizure in patients with sarcoidosis is often difficult to control, and treatment requires both antiepileptic drugs and glucocorticoids to address the underlying abnormality.[26,27] Approximately 20% of patients with neurosarcoidosis exhibit signs and symptoms of cognitive and behavioral problems.[14] The cause of these manifestations is likely multifactorial in nature, including encephalopathy from neurosarcoidosis itself, use of glucocorticoids, and the emotional burden of living with a chronic disease that could be organ and life threatening.[26] A cross-sectional study of 154 patients with sarcoidosis found that up to 60% of patients suffered from depression.[28]

The pathogenesis of encephalopathy associated with neurosarcoidosis remains poorly understood. Findings consistent with diffuse parenchymal inflammation are detectable on imaging studies.[29,30] Histopathologic evidence of granulomatous cerebral angiitis in patients with neurosarcoidosis may be seen on biopsy of brain tissues and may also predispose patients to cerebrovascular accident (CVA).[31,32] In fact, a recent population-based study has demonstrated that the risk of CVA among patients with sarcoidosis was 3 times higher than the general population. Nonetheless, premature atherosclerosis associated with chronic inflammation from sarcoidosis is probably the major factor for CVA, because patients with sarcoidosis are at increased risk of other atherosclerotic diseases, such as myocardial infarction and peripheral arterial disease.[33]

Intracranial granulomatous mass lesions can be seen in any part of the central nervous system (CNS) and can present as a solitary mass or multiple nodules.[14,15] These mass lesions can cause focal neurologic deficit, seizure, and symptoms of increased intracranial pressure.[15] Diagnosis is often challenging because several other diseases can cause intracranial mass lesions, such as infection and tumor. Thus, biopsy is generally required to establish the diagnosis of neurosarcoidosis, although the sensitivity of brain parenchymal biopsy to demonstrate noncaseating granuloma is only 60%.[23]

Neuroendocrinologic Dysfunction

Granulomas infiltration of the pituitary gland and hypothalamus is seen in 2% to 8% of patients with neurosarcoidosis.[13,17,20,21] Polydipsia and polyuria as a result of diabetes insipidus are the most common clinical presentations, followed by signs and symptoms of hyperprolactinemia (amenorrhea, galactorrhea, and decreased libido) as a result of hypothalamic dysfunction.[22,34] Interestingly, a study of 80 patients with sarcoidosis without any clinical manifestation of neuroendocrinologic dysfunction reported hyperprolactinemia in 15% of the cases.[35] Other hypothalamus-pituitary hormonal axes, including thyroid hormone, growth hormone, and cortisol, could be affected as well.[15,26,34] Rare manifestations of hypothalamic sarcoidosis include hyperphagia and obesity due to satiety center involvement,[36,37] extreme variations of body temperature due to involvement of body temperature regulator,[38] insomnia, and personality changes.[39]

Spinal Cord Disease

Spinal cord sarcoidosis was once thought to be rare and account for less than 5% of neurosarcoidosis cases.[11,15,20] However, more recent studies report spinal cord involvement in up to 20% of these cases.[14,18,22] Sarcoidal granulomas can be found in intramedullary, intradural, and extradural portions of the spinal cord and have a predilection for thoracic and cervical spinal cord.[26,40,41] Subacute to chronic onset of paresthesia and weakness below the affected spinal cord level are the most common presentations.[40,41] Other manifestations include back pain, radicular pain, proprioceptive disturbance, sphincter dysfunction, and cauda equina syndrome.[15,40–42] Historically, outcome of patients with spinal cord involvement was unfavorable with high incidence of permanent neurologic deficit.[15] However, recent case series have demonstrated a more favorable functional outcome, possibly because of a more prompt recognition and aggressive glucocorticoid and immunosuppressive therapy.[41,43]

Peripheral Neuropathy

The prevalence of peripheral neuropathy among patients with neurosarcoidosis is between 2% and 6%.[15,17,20] Reported patterns of large-fiber neuropathy include mononeuropathy, polyradiculopathy, Guillain-Barré syndrome, and symmetric distal polyneuropathy, which could be sensorimotor, mostly motor, or mostly sensory.[26,44–47] Small fiber neuropathy causing chronic pain and paresthesia is also seen in patients with sarcoidosis.[26,44,48] Epineural and perineural granulomatous inflammation and granulomatous vasculitis can be seen on nerve biopsy and are thought to be the underlying pathogenesis of the axonal injury.[44,49] Prognosis of peripheral neuropathy appears to be more benign than other types of neurosarcoidosis because most patients respond favorably to glucocorticoids therapy.[12,13]

DIAGNOSTIC TESTS

Similar to systemic sarcoidosis, diagnosis of neurosarcoidosis requires the presence of noncaseating granuloma and compatible clinical presentations after exclusion of alternative diagnoses.[50] The presence of noncaseating granuloma itself is not sufficient to make a definite diagnosis because it could be seen in other conditions, such as foreign body reaction, tuberculosis, and fungal infection.[11,25]

Given the invasive nature of biopsy of the nervous system, histopathologic confirmation is often not feasible. In addition, false negative results are common, with up to 30% to 40% of brain parenchymal and meningeal biopsies failing to confirm the diagnosis.[23] Zajicek and colleagues[21] proposed set criteria for diagnosis of neurosarcoidosis that defines "possible" and "probable" diagnosis using diagnostic tests without histopathology (**Table 2**).

Neuroimaging

Brain and spin MRI are the most sensitive imaging modalities to detect abnormalities in the brain parenchyma, leptomeninges, dura mater, and spinal cord.[51] However, the

Table 2
Proposed diagnostic criteria for neurosarcoidosis

	Definition
Definite	Suggestive clinical presentation of neurosarcoidosis *Plus* Positive histopathology from nervous system biopsy *Plus* Exclusion of other diseases
Probable	Suggestive clinical presentation of neurosarcoidosis *Plus* Evidence of inflammation in the CNS[a] *Plus* Evidence of systemic sarcoidosis[b] *Plus* Exclusion of other diseases
Possible	Suggestive clinical presentation of neurosarcoidosis with exclusion of other diseases whereby the criteria for definite and probable neurosarcoidosis are not met

[a] Evidence of inflammation in CNS includes elevated protein and/or cells in CSF, the presence of oligoclonal band, and abnormal brain MRI.
[b] Evidence of systemic sarcoidosis includes positive histopathology from extraneural organ and/or at least 2 indirect pieces of evidence from gallium scan, chest imaging, and ACE.
Adapted from Zajicek JP, Scolding NJ, Foster O, et al. Central nervous system sarcoidosis – diagnosis and management. QJM 1999;92:103–17.

sensitivity of these tests is significantly reduced after glucocorticoids exposure, and they are not sensitive for cranial neuropathy.[11,17]

Brain parenchymal abnormalities are seen on MRI in more than half of patients with neurosarcoidosis.[14,21] Multiple nonenhancing periventricular white matter lesions are the most common abnormalities.[21,51,52] However, the lesions are nonspecific and could also be seen in multiple sclerosis and vasculopathy.[11,51] Enhancing intraparenchymal mass or nodular lesions are also seen and are often mistaken for tumor or demyelinating disease (**Figs. 1** and **2**).[51,52] Central necrosis is uncommon. Patients with enhancing intraparenchymal mass lesions often present with seizure.[53]

The reported prevalence of leptomeningeal involvement among patients with neurosarcoidosis varied from 15% to 70%.[53–55] The variability is in part due to different MRI techniques used in each study because leptomeningeal sarcoidosis is best seen with contrast-enhanced T1-weighted images.[11,56,57] Diffuse or nodular enhancement of the leptomeninges with predilection for suprasellar and frontal basal meninges is the typical MRI finding (**Fig. 3**).[11,25,51] Leptomeningeal enhancement around hypothalamus and pituitary stalk is common and could be seen in isolation or in association with involvement of basal leptomeninges.[51,53] Basal meningeal involvement is not specific for neurosarcoidosis because it can be seen in several conditions, such as tuberculosis, meningeal carcinomatosis, and granulomatosis with polyangiitis.[11,51]

Dural involvement by sarcoidosis can present as focal masses or diffuse dural thickening that enhances homogenously on contrast-enhanced T1-weighted images but are hypointense on T1-weighted images.[11,52] These findings can mimic meningioma and dural metastases. Dural disease can be distinguished from leptomeningeal disease by the lack of involvement of the cortical sulci and the cistern around the base of the brain.[51]

Typical MRI findings of cranial neuropathy include enlargement and enhancement of the affected cranial nerve on contrast-enhanced T1-weighted

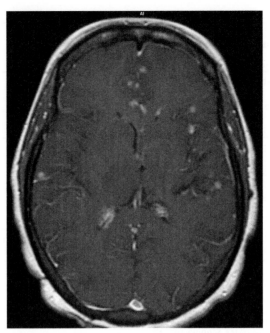

Fig. 1. Axial contrast-enhanced T1-weighted MRI demonstrates multiple intracerebral-enhancing nodular lesions.

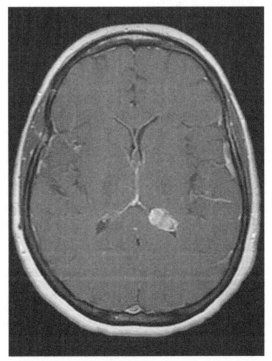

Fig. 2. Axial contrast-enhanced T1-weighted MRI demonstrates a solitary enhancing mass lesion within the posterior horn of the left lateral ventricle.

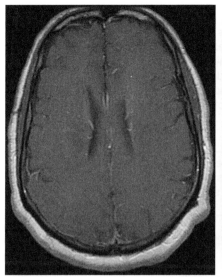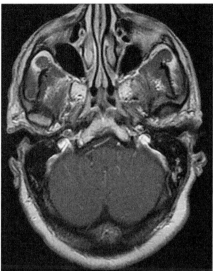

Fig. 3. Axial contrast-enhanced T1-weighted MRI demonstrates diffuse enhancement of leptomeninges in both cerebral and cerebellar hemispheres.

images.[51,53] However, clinical signs and symptoms of cranial neuropathy have a poor correlation with MRI abnormalities because some patients had abnormal MRI without any clinical symptoms, whereas others have clinical symptoms with normal MRI.[51–53] External compression of cranial nerve from dural/leptomeningeal disease or sinonasal inflammation/mass can cause cranial neuropathy as well.[11,51]

Involvement of spinal cord by neurosarcoidosis is usually a result of spinal cord and/or spinal nerve root compression by granulomatous inflammation/nodules of the leptomeninges best visualized on contrast-enhanced T1-weighted images, similar to sarcoidosis of the intracranial leptomeninges.[51] Intramedullary spinal lesions are rare and account for less than 5% of neurosarcoidosis.[14,15,17]

Cerebrospinal Fluid Analysis

CSF analysis may show evidence of CNS inflammation with pleocytosis, high protein content, and sometimes low glucose concentration, particularly in cases of meningeal and brain parenchymal involvement.[14,17,26] The CSF profile is not specific for sarcoidosis and can be seen in viral meningitis and other noninfectious inflammatory diseases of the CNS, such as systemic lupus erythematosus.[44] In addition, CSF analysis is usually normal for patients with isolated cranial neuropathy.[15] Therefore, CSF analysis is more useful to exclude other diseases (such as infectious meningitis and meningeal carcinomatosis) rather than to confirm the diagnosis of neurosarcoidosis.

The diagnostic utility of CSF angiotensin-converting enzyme (ACE) levels for diagnosis of neurosarcoidosis is limited because the levels can be elevated in numerous conditions such as multiple sclerosis, brain tumor, and Alzheimer disease.[11] Two large studies found that only 33% to 50% of patients who had elevated CSF ACE levels had neurosarcoidosis and 5% to 7% of those who did not have neurosarcoidosis had elevated CSF ACE levels.[58,59] To the poor performance of serum ACE levels for diagnosis of systemic sarcoidosis with high false positive and negative rate.[60]

TREATMENTS

Unlike pulmonary sarcoidosis, spontaneous resolution of neurosarcoidosis is uncommon (except for facial nerve palsy), and treatment is generally indicated to minimize morbidity and mortality.[6] Unfortunately, there have been no randomized, placebo-controlled trials in neurosarcoidosis to guide treatment. Therefore, all recommendations are based on clinical experience and limited data from observation studies. Doses, adverse reactions, and monitoring of the commonly used medications in neurosarcoidosis are summarized in **Table 3**.

Glucocorticoids

Glucocorticoids are the cornerstone for the treatment of neurosarcoidosis. Their efficacy for the treatment of neurosarcoidosis has been shown in several observational studies, although the response rate seems to be lower than pulmonary

Table 3
Medications commonly used for treatment of neurosarcoidosis

Medication	Dose	Common Adverse Effects	Monitoring
Glucocorticoids			
Prednisone or prednisolone	Initially 0.5–1.0 mg/kg/d oral with slow taper	Hyperglycemia, hypertension, weight gain, mood change, psychosis, insomnia, osteoporosis, GI upset, cataract, infection, adrenal insufficiency	Blood pressure, blood glucose
Methylprednisolone	1000 mg IV daily for 3–5 d	Same as prednisone	Same as prednisone
Immunosuppressive agent			
Methotrexate	10–25 mg oral or SC weekly	Hepatitis, cytopenia, pneumonitis, infection, GI upset, teratogenicity	CBC, LFT, creatinine
Cyclophosphamide	0.6–1.0 g/m² IV q4 wk or 1.5–2.0 mg/kg/d oral	Hepatitis, cytopenia, infection, hemorrhagic cystitis, infertility, cardiac toxicity	CBC, LFT, creatinine, urinalysis
Chloroquine	500–750 mg oral daily	Retinal toxicity, tinnitus, hearing loss, drug rash	Ophthalmologic examination
Hydroxychloroquine	200–400 mg oral daily or divided into 2 times per day	Retinal toxicity, tinnitus, hearing loss, drug rash	Ophthalmologic examination
Biologic agent			
Infliximab	3–5 mg/kg IV at 0, 2, and 6 wk for induction, then every 4–8 wk for maintenance	Infusion reaction, infection, cytopenia, exacerbation of congestive heart failure, demyelinating disease	CBC

Abbreviations: CBC, complete blood count; GI, gastrointestinal; IV, intravenous; LFT, liver function test; SC, subcutaneous.

sarcoidosis.[14,15,20,21,24] Different glucocorticoid regimens have been used for different types of neurosarcoidosis. Initial dosing of prednisone equivalent 1.0 mg/kg/d is generally required for central abnormalities, including meningitis, intraparenchymal brain lesions, encephalopathy, and intramedullary spinal cord lesions. Prednisone 0.5 mg/kg/d may be sufficient for cranial neuropathy and peripheral neuropathy. Patients who do not respond to high-dose oral prednisone or who have a rapidly progressive disease course may benefit from a 3- to 5-day course of intravenous methylprednisolone at 1000 mg/d.[61,62] Once adequate response is achieved, gradual glucocorticoid taper can be undertaken within 4 to 8 weeks. In general, patients with neurosarcoidosis require a prolonged course of glucocorticoids therapy (at least 6–12 months)[23,26] except for facial nerve palsy that may need only 4 to 6 weeks of therapy.[18,20,63]

Immunosuppressive Agents

Patients with neurosarcoidosis usually have a good response to high-dose glucocorticoids.[12] However, some patients do not tolerate the adverse effects associated with high-dose initial or protracted lower-dose treatment. In addition, relapse tends to occur when the dose of glucocorticoids is reduced to lower than 20 to 25 mg of prednisone equivalent.[21] Thus, immunosuppressive agents are often required as second-line therapy. Some experts advocate use of combination therapy for glucocorticoids and immunosuppressive agents as initial therapy, although this approach is controversial because it is associated with a higher risk of infection and other adverse effects.[64]

Methotrexate, a folic acid analogue, is the immunosuppressive agent for which there are the most extensive efficacy data for neurosarcoidosis. One study observed that 17 out of 28 patients (61%) who had failed glucocorticoids therapy had a good response to methotrexate.[20] Another case report described 2 patients with progressive disease despite treatment with glucocorticoids who responded well to methotrexate as second-line therapy.[24] The doses of methotrexate used in the reported patients range from 10 mg per week to 25 mg per week. Adverse effects of methotrexate do not occur frequently and can be lessened by use of folic acid (see **Table 2**).[65]

Cyclophosphamide is an alkylating agent that has been used extensively in autoimmune diseases. Data on its efficacy in neurosarcoidosis are largely drawn from case reports and case series. One case series found that 4 of 10 patients who did not respond to either glucocorticoids or methotrexate responded well to intravenous cyclophosphamide (500 mg to 700 mg every 2 weeks) with objective improvement by MRI and/or CSF analysis.[20] Another study of 7 patients with glucocorticoids-refractory neurosarcoidosis who were subsequently treated with intravenous cyclophosphamide (500 mg to 1000 mg every 3 weeks) found that 4 patients (57%) had clinical improvement.[66] Adverse effects of cyclophosphamide are more frequent and serious than methotrexate.

Chloroquine and hydroxychloroquine are 2 antimalarial drugs that have been used in treatment connective tissue diseases and inflammatory arthritis. Their efficacy for cutaneous sarcoidosis is well established, but data on their use in neurosarcoidosis are relatively limited.[67,68] A series of 12 patients who could not tolerate or did not wish to take glucocorticoids were treated with chloroquine or hydroxychloroquine monotherapy with stabilization and/or improvement of neurologic symptoms in 10 (83%) patients.[69]

Data on other immunosuppressive agents, including mycophenolate mofetil, azathioprine, and thalidomide, are even more scarce and limited to few case reports. These medications are considered the third-line therapy and are generally used when the more established medications fail to help improve or stabilize the disease.[17,70–73]

Biologic Agents

Infliximab is a chimeric monoclonal antibody against tumor-necrosis factor-alpha that is an important cytokine for granuloma formation.[74] Randomized controlled trials of infliximab for pulmonary sarcoidosis demonstrated improvement of pulmonary function tests compared with placebo.[75,76] Infliximab also appears to be effective for patients with neurosarcoidosis who have failed other therapies based on several case reports and case series.[77–79] For example, a series of 18 patients with glucocorticoid and/or immunosuppressive agents–refractory neurosarcoidosis treated with infliximab reported significant clinical improvement in 16 (89%) of these patients.[79]

Data on other biologic agents are very scarce with only few reported cases of neurosarcoidosis successfully treated with adalimumab and rituximab.[80,81]

SUMMARY

Neurosarcoidosis is an uncommon manifestation of sarcoidosis that is associated with significant morbidity and mortality. Diagnosis of neurosarcoidosis is often challenging, because clinical manifestations and findings on imaging studies can be mimicked by several other diseases. Glucocorticoids are the cornerstone for the treatment of neurosarcoidosis; immunosuppressive agents are also often required. Clinical trials are needed to establish the efficacy of these treatments.

REFERENCES

1. Chen ES, Moller DR. Etiology of sarcoidosis. Clin Chest Med 2008;29:365–77.
2. Brito-Zeron P, Sellares J, Bosch X, et al. Epidemiologic patterns of disease expression in sarcoidosis: age, gender and ethnicity-related differences. Clin Exp Rheumatol 2016;34:380–8.
3. Morimoto T, Azuma A, Abe S, et al. Epidemiology of sarcoidosis in Japan. Eur Respir J 2008;31:372–9.
4. Cozier YC, Berman JS, Palmer JR, et al. Sarcoidosis in black women in the United States: data from the black women's health study. Chest 2011;139:144–50.
5. Ungprasert P, Carmona EM, Utz JP, et al. Epidemiology of sarcoidosis 1946-2013: a population-based study. Mayo Clin Proc 2016;191:183–8.
6. Judson MA, Boan AD, Lackland DT. The clinical course of sarcoidosis: presentation, diagnosis, and treatment in a large white and black cohort in the United States. Sarcoidosis Vasc Diffuse Lung Dis 2012;29:119–27.
7. Baughman RP, Teirstein AS, Judson MA, et al, Case Control Etiologic Study of Sarcoidosis (ACCESS) Research Group. Clinical characteristics of patients in a case control study of sarcoidosis. Am J Respir Crit Care Med 2001;164:1885–9.
8. Sharma SK, Mohan A, Guleria JS. Clinical characteristics, pulmonary function abnormalities and outcome of prednisolone treatment in 106 patients with sarcoidosis. J Assoc Physicians India 2001;49:697–704.
9. Iwai K, Tachibana T, Takemura T, et al. Pathological studies on sarcoidosis autopsy. Acta Pathol Jpn 1993;43:372–6.
10. Ricker W, Clark M. Sarcoidosis; a clinicopathological review of 300 cases, including 22 autopsies. Am J Clin Pathol 1949;19:725–49.
11. Nozaki K, Judson MA. Neurosarcoidosis: clinical manifestations, diagnosis and treatment. Presse Med 2012;41:e331–48.

12. Allen RKA, Sellars RE, Sandstrom PA. A prospective study of 32 patients with neurosarcoidosis. Sarcoidosis Vasc Diffuse Lung Dis 2003;20:118–25.
13. Ferriby D, de Seze J, Stojkovic T, et al. Long-term follow-up of neurosarcoidosis. Neurology 2001;57:927–9.
14. Joseph FG, Scolding NJ. Neurosarcoidosis: a study of 30 new cases. J Neurol Neurosurg Psychiatry 2009;80:297–304.
15. Stern BJ, Krumholz A, Johns C, et al. Sarcoidosis and its neurological manifestations. Arch Neurol 1985;42:909–17.
16. Carlson ML, White JR, Espahbodi M, et al. Cranial base manifestation of neurosarcoidosis: a review of 305 patients. Otol Neurotol 2014;36:156–66.
17. Pawate S, Moses H, Sriram S. Presentations and outcomes of neurosarcoidosis: a study of 54 cases. QJM 2009;102:449–60.
18. Dua A, Manadan A. Images in clinical medicine. Heerfordt's syndrome, or uveoparotid fever. N Engl J Med 2013;369:458.
19. Ungprasert P, Crowson CS, Matteson EL. Clinical characteristics of parotid gland sarcoidosis: a population-based study. JAMA Otolaryngol Head Neck Surg 2016; 142:503–4.
20. Lower EE, Broderick JP, Brott TG, et al. Diagnosis and management of neurological sarcoidosis. Arch Intern Med 1997;157:1864–8.
21. Zajicek JP, Scolding NJ, Foster O, et al. Central nervous system sarcoidosis – diagnosis and management. QJM 1999;92:103–17.
22. Kane K. Deafness in sarcoidosis. J Laryngol Otol 1976;90:531–7.
23. Stern BJ, Aksamit A, Clifford D, et al. Neurologic presentation of sarcoidosis. Neurol Clin 2010;28:185–98.
24. Marangoni S, Argentiero V, Tavolato B. Neurosarcoidosis. Clinical description of 7 cases with proposal for a new diagnostic strategy. J Neurol 2006;253:488–95.
25. Nowak DA, Widenka DC. Neurosarcoidosis: a review of its intracranial manifestation. J Neurol 2001;248:363–72.
26. Terushkin V, Stern BJ, Judson MA, et al. Neurosarcoidosis. Presentations and management. Neurologist 2010;16:2–15.
27. Krumholz A, Stern BJ, Stern EG. Clinical implications of seizures in neurosarcoidosis. Arch Neurol 1991;48:842–4.
28. Chang B, Steimel J, Moller DR, et al. Depression in sarcoidosis. Am J Respir Crit Care Med 2001;163:329–34.
29. Brook J Jr, Strickland MC, William JP, et al. Computed tomography changes in neurosarcoidosis clearing with steroid treatment. J Comput Assist Tomogr 1979;3:398–9.
30. Ho SU, Berenberg RA, Kim KS, et al. Sarcoid encephalopathy with diffuse inflammation and focal hydrocephalus shown by sequential CT. Neurology 1979;29: 1161–5.
31. Herring AB, Urich H. Sarcoidosis of the central nervous system. J Neurol Sci 1969;9:405–22.
32. Meyer JS, Foley JM, Campagna-Pinto D. Granulomatous angiitis of the meninges in sarcoidosis. Arch Neurol 1953;69:587–600.
33. Ungprasert P, Crowson CS, Matteson EL. Risk of cardiovascular disease among patients with sarcoidosis: a population-based retrospective cohort study, 1976-2013. Eur Respir J 2017;49:1601290.
34. Langrand C, Bihan H, Raverot G. Hypothalami-pituitary sarcoidosis: a multicenter study of 24 patients. QJM 2012;105:981–95.
35. Nacho K, Noma K, Sato B, et al. Serum prolactin levels in eighty patients with sarcoidosis. Eur J Clin Invest 1978;8:37–40.

36. Vesely DL. Hypothalamic sarcoidosis: a new cause of morbid obesity. South Med J 1989;82:758–61.
37. Vanhoof J, Wilms G, Bouillon R. Hypothalamic hypopituitarism with hyperphagia and subacute dementia due to neurosarcoidosis: case report and literature review. Acta Clin Belg 1992;47:319–28.
38. Jefferson M. Sarcoidosis of the nervous system. Brain 1957;80:540–56.
39. Gjerse A, Kjerulif-Jensen K. Hypothalamic lesion caused by Boeck's sarcoidosis. J Clin Endocrinol Metab 1950;10:1602–8.
40. Cohen-Aubert F, Galanaud D, Grabli D, et al. Spinal cord sarcoidosis. Clinical and laboratory profile and outcome of 31 patients in a case-control study. Medicine 2010;89:133–40.
41. Bradley DA, Lower EE, Baughman RP. Diagnosis and management of spinal sarcoidosis. Sarcoidosis Vasc Diffuse Lung Dis 2006;23:58–65.
42. Ku A, Lachmann E, Tunnel R, et al. Neurosarcoidosis of the conus medullar is and cauda equina presenting as paraparesis: case report and literature review. Paraplegia 1996;34:116–20.
43. Durel CA, Marignier R, Maucort-Boulch D, et al. Clinical features and prognostic factors of spinal cord sarcoidosis: a multicenter observational study of 20 BIOPSY-PROVEN patients. J Neurol 2016;263:981–90.
44. Hoitsma E, Faber CG, Drent M, et al. Neurosarcoidosis: a clinical dilemma. Lancet Neurol 2004;3:397–407.
45. Koffman B, Junck L, Elias SB, et al. Polyradiculopathy in sarcoidosis. Muscle Nerve 1999;22:608–13.
46. Nemni R, Galassi G, Cohen M, et al. Symmetric sarcoid polyneuropathy: analysis of a sural nerve biopsy. Neurology 1981;31:1217–23.
47. Miller R, Sheron N, Semple S. Sarcoidosis presenting with an acute Guillain-Barre syndrome. Postgrad Med J 1989;65:765–7.
48. Tavee JO, Karwa K, Ahmed Z, et al. Sarcoidosis-associated small fiber neuropathy in a large cohort: clinical aspects and response to IVIG and anti-TNF alpha treatment. Respir Med 2017;126:135–8.
49. Said G, Lacroix C, Plante-Bordeneuve V, et al. Nerve granulomas and vasculitis in sarcoid peripheral neuropathy: a clinicopathological study of 11 patients. Brain 2002;125:264–75.
50. Costabel U, Hunninghake GW. ATS/ERS/WASOG statement on sarcoidosis. Sarcoidosis statement committee. American Thoracic Society. European Respiratory Society. World Association for Sarcoidosis and Other Granulomatous Disorders. Eur Respir J 1999;14:735–7.
51. Smith JK, Matheus MG, Castillo M. Imaging manifestations of neurosarcoidosis. AJR Am J Roentgenol 2004;182:289–95.
52. Dumas JL, Valeyre D, Chapelon-Abric C, et al. Central nervous system sarcoidosis: follow-up at MRI during steroid therapy. Radiology 2000;214:411–20.
53. Christofordis GA, Spickler EM, Reccio MV, et al. MR of CNS sarcoidosis: correlation of imaging features to clinical symptoms and response to treatment. AJNR Am J Neuroradiol 1999;20:655–69.
54. Lexa FJ, Grossman RI. MR of sarcoidosis in the head and spine: spectrum of manifestations and radiographic response to steroid therapy. AJNR Am J Neuroradiol 1994;15:973–82.
55. Fels C, Riegel A, Javaheripour-Otto K, et al. Neurosarcoidosis. Findings in MRI. Clin Imaging 2004;28:166–9.
56. Sherman JL, Stern BJ. Sarcoidosis of the CNS: comparison of unenhanced and enhanced MR images. AJR Am J Roentgenol 1990;155:1293–301.

57. Hashmi M, Kyristsis AP. Diagnosis and treatment of intramedullary spinal cord sarcoidosis. J Neurol 1998;245:178–85.
58. Tahmoush AJ, Albert J. CSF-ACE activity in probable CNS neurosarcoidosis. Sarcoidosis Vasc Diffuse Lung Dis 2002;19:191–7.
59. Dale JC, O'Brien JF. Determination of angiotensin-converting enzyme levels in cerebrospinal fluid is not useful test for the diagnosis of neurosarcoidosis. Mayo Clin Proc 1999;74:535.
60. Ungprasert P, Carmona EM, Crowson CS, et al. Diagnostic utility of angiotensin-converting enzyme in sarcoidosis: a population-based retrospective cohort study. Lung 2016;194:91–5.
61. Adamec I, Ozretic D, Zadro I, et al. Progressive meningoencephalitis due to neurosarcoidosis. Clin Neurol Neurosurg 2013;115:793–5.
62. Lally E, Murchison AP, Moster ML. Compressive optic neuropathy from neurosarcoidosis. Ophthal Plast Reconstr Surg 2015;31:e79.
63. Tamme T, Liebur E, Kulla A. Sarcoidosis (Heerfordt syndrome): a case report. Stoxmatologija 2007;9:61–4.
64. Youssef J, Novosad SA, Winthrop KL. Infection risk and safety of corticosteroid use. Rheum Dis Clin North Am 2016;42:157–76.
65. Romão VC, Lima A, Bernardes M, et al. Three decades of low-dose methotrexate in rheumatoid arthritis: can we predict toxicity? Immunol Res 2014;60(2–3):289–310.
66. Doty JD, Mazur JE, Judson MA. Treatment of corticosteroid-resistant neurosarcoidosis with a short-course cyclophosphamide regimen. Chest 2003;124:2023–6.
67. Ungprasert P, Wetter DA, Crowson CS, et al. Epidemiology of cutaneous sarcoidosis, 1976-2013: a population based study from Olmsted County, Minnesota. J Eur Acad Dermatol Venereol 2016;30:1799–804.
68. Wanat KA, Rosenbach M. A practical approach to cutaneous sarcoidosis. Am J Clin Dermatol 2014;15:283–97.
69. Sharma OP. Effectiveness of chloroquine and hydroxychloroquine in treating selected patients with sarcoidosis with neurological involvement. Arch Neurol 1998;55:1248–54.
70. Hammond ER, Kaplin AI, Kerr DA. Thalidomide for acute treatment of neurosarcoidosis. Spinal Cord 2007;45:802–3.
71. Chaussenot A, Bourg V, Chanalet S, et al. Neurosarcoidosis treated with mycophenilate mofetil: two cases. Rev Neurol 2007;163:471–5.
72. Corbett J. Treating CNS sarcoidosis with infliximab and mycophenolate mofetil. Curr Neurol Neurosci Rep 2009;9:339–40.
73. Androdias G, Maillet D, Marignier R, et al. Mycophenolate mofetil may be effective in CNS sarcoidosis but not in sarcoid myopathy. Neurology 2011;76:1168–72.
74. Amber KT, Bloom R, Mrowietz U, et al. TNF-alpha: a treatment target or causes of sarcoidosis? J Eur Acad Dermatol Venereol 2015;29:2104–11.
75. Baughman RP, Drent M, Kavuru K, et al. Infliximab therapy in patients with chronic sarcoidosis and pulmonary involvement. Am J Respir Crit Care Med 2006;174:795–802.
76. Rossman MD, Newman LS, Baughman RP, et al. A double-blinded, randomized, placebo-controlled trial of infliximab in subjects with active pulmonary sarcoidosis. Sarcoidosis Vasc Diffuse Lung Dis 2006;23:201–8.
77. Sodhi M, Pearson K, White ES, et al. Infliximab therapy rescues cyclophosphamide failure in severe central nervous system sarcoidosis. Respir Med 2009;103:268–73.

78. Toth C, Martin L, Morrish W, et al. Dramatic MRI improvement with refractory neurosarcoidosis treated with infliximab. Acta Neurol Scand 2007;116:259–62.
79. Aubart FC, Bouvry D, Galanaud D, et al. Long-term outcomes of refractory neurosarcoidosis treated with infliximab. J Neurol 2017;264(5):891–7.
80. Marnane M, Lynch T, Scott J, et al. Steroid-unresponsive neurosarcoidosis successfully treated with adalimumab. J Neurol 2009;256:139–40.
81. Bomprezzi R, Pati S, Chansakul C, et al. A case of neurosarcoidosis successfully treated with rituximab. Neurology 2010;75:568–70.

Central Nervous System Infections Associated with Immunosuppressive Therapy for Rheumatic Disease

Michael J. Bradshaw, MD[a], Tracey A. Cho, MD, MA[b], Felicia C. Chow, MD, MAS[c],*

KEYWORDS

- Central nervous system infection • Immunosuppression
- Immunomodulatory therapy • Rheumatic disease

KEY POINTS

- Rheumatologists should be familiar with central nervous system (CNS) infections associated with immunosuppressive therapy, and changes in neurologic function should be queried at every clinic visit.
- The risk of infection associated with glucocorticoids increases with dose and duration of therapy, and combination regimens likely compound the risk of infection.
- Although few data suggest increased risk of CNS infection from methotrexate, rheumatologists should be familiar with the neurotoxic side effects that can develop.
- Tumor necrosis factor inhibitors increase the risk of granulomatous and bacterial infections and can also cause idiopathic granulomatous or demyelinating reactions.
- Rituximab is associated with rare cases of progressive multifocal leukoencephalopathy; patients should be carefully monitored clinically and clinicians should maintain a high index of suspicion.

INTRODUCTION

The risk of opportunistic infections and pathogens that can cause disease in healthy hosts is heightened in patients with rheumatologic conditions treated with immunosuppressive and immunomodulatory agents.[1] In addition, immune dysregulation

Disclosures: The authors have no disclosures to report.
Funding: This work was supported by NIH/NCATS KL2TR000143 (F.C. Chow).
[a] Partners Multiple Sclerosis Center, Brigham and Women's Hospital and Massachusetts General Hospital, 60 Fenwood Road, 4th floor, Boston, MA 02115, USA; [b] Department of Neurology, Massachusetts General Hospital, 55 Fruit Street, Boston, MA 02114, USA; [c] Department of Neurology and Division of Infectious Diseases, University of California, San Francisco, Zuckerberg San Francisco General Hospital, 1001 Potrero Avenue, Building 1, Room 101, San Francisco, CA 94110, USA
* Corresponding author.
E-mail address: felicia.chow@ucsf.edu

Rheum Dis Clin N Am 43 (2017) 607–619
http://dx.doi.org/10.1016/j.rdc.2017.06.009
rheumatic.theclinics.com

associated with underlying rheumatic disease may predispose to infectious complications. Infections of the central nervous system (CNS) are particularly important to recognize given high associated morbidity and mortality and the complexity of distinguishing between CNS infections and neurologic manifestations of rheumatic disease. This article first presents 2 illustrative cases followed by a discussion of a selection of commonly used agents in the treatment of rheumatic disease and the risk of CNS infections associated with their use.

Case 1

A 25-year-old woman with systemic lupus erythematosus (SLE) presented with 3 weeks of headache, photosensitivity, and vomiting. Her SLE had been treated with varying doses of prednisone, up to 50 mg daily, and azathioprine 200 mg daily. Lumbar puncture showed normal opening pressure. She had a moderate lymphocyte-predominant pleocytosis, mildly increased protein, and normal glucose. Cryptococcal antigen was positive in the serum and cerebrospinal fluid (CSF). She was treated with intravenous amphotericin B liposomal and flucytosine followed by oral fluconazole with complete resolution of her symptoms. She has continued on maintenance fluconazole while on immunosuppression for active SLE.

Case 2

A 61-year-old woman with rheumatoid arthritis (RA) presented with headaches, vertigo, and painful paresthesias on the trunk. A brain and spine MRI scan with contrast showed diffuse ring-enhancing lesions (**Fig. 1**). She had most recently been treated

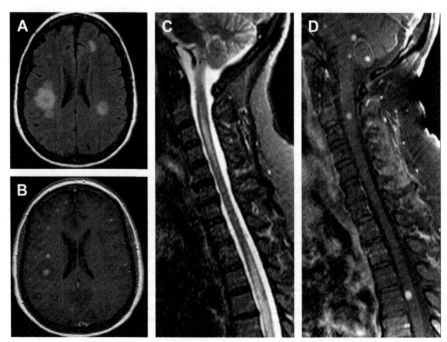

Fig. 1. Histoplasma encephalomyelitis in the setting of prior rituximab and methotrexate use. (*A*) Axial T2-FLAIR (fluid-attenuated inversion recovery) brain MRI, (*B*) axial T1 postcontrast brain MRI, (*C*) midsagittal T2 MRI of the spine, (*D*) axial T1 postcontrast MRI of the spine.

with rituximab and methotrexate (MTX), which were discontinued 1 year before presentation consequent to frequent infections. She had also received glucocorticoids, etanercept, and adalimumab. Lumbar puncture showed no white blood cells, mildly increased protein, and normal glucose. Serum and urine *Histoplasma* antigen were positive. She was treated with intravenous amphotericin B liposomal followed by itraconazole for CNS histoplasmosis. She improved clinically with resolution of lesions.

Broadly Immunosuppressive Agents

Glucocorticoids

Glucocorticoids bind to their specific intracellular receptors, leading to downregulation of the inflammatory response through a broad range of mechanisms.[2–5] Innate immunity is inhibited by depletion of immune cells, impaired migration and phagocytosis, and decreased production of inflammatory cytokines.[6] Adaptive immune function is attenuated through reduction in the number and function of T and B cells.[7–9] Suppression of innate and adaptive immunity associated with glucocorticoid use increases the risk for virtually all types of infections, many of which can affect the CNS, including pyogenic and intracellular bacteria (eg, *Staphylococcus*, *Salmonella*), mycobacteria (eg, *Mycobacterium tuberculosis*), fungi (eg, *Cryptococcus*, *Candida*), viruses (eg, herpes viruses), and parasites (eg, *Toxoplasma gondii*, *Strongyloides*).[10] *Listeria* and *Nocardia* species are examples of pathogens with a predilection for the CNS for which glucocorticoid use is a major risk factor.

The risk of infection associated with glucocorticoid use increases with higher dosing and longer duration of therapy, along with patient-specific factors including older age, lower functional status, and underlying illness.[11–15] A meta-analysis of 71 clinical trials found that the overall rate of infections was higher among patients on glucocorticoid therapy than placebo (relative risk, 1.6; 95% confidence interval [CI], 1.3–1.9). However, infection rates were not increased in patients taking less than 10 prednisone-equivalent milligrams daily or a cumulative dose of 700 mg. Glucocorticoids used in combination with other immunosuppressants confer greater risk of systemic and CNS infections, particularly at higher cumulative doses (see case 1).[16] In one series of 23 patients with SLE diagnosed with a CNS infection, all were on prednisone doses of 20 to 60 mg/d, with an average dose of 29 mg. Nearly half of patients had recently received pulse cyclophosphamide, and 2 were on mycophenolate mofetil.[17]

In order to reduce risk of infection, the lowest dose of glucocorticoids should be used for the shortest duration, and concurrent use of other immunosuppression should be avoided when possible. Alternate-day dosing of short-acting glucocorticoids has been suggested to reduce associated risks, although evidence of decreased infectious complications is debatable.[18–20] Glucocorticoid dose reduction or discontinuation should be considered while treating infectious complications. Although prophylaxis against infections such as *Pneumocystis jiroveci* pneumonia for patients requiring long-term glucocorticoid use (eg, the equivalent of 20 mg/d or more of prednisone for a minimum of 1 month) is common practice and can have activity against some CNS pathogens (eg, *Listeria*, *Nocardia*), no data are available regarding the utility of prophylaxis for CNS infections. Clinicians should refer to guidelines regarding the timing of vaccinations for patients on glucocorticoids, because deferral, particularly for live attenuated vaccines (eg, herpes zoster vaccine), may be required for patients on higher doses.[21]

Methotrexate

MTX inhibits dihydrofolate reductase and is a mainstay of treatment of RA and other rheumatic conditions. Current evidence points to adenosine signaling as a primary driver of the antiinflammatory effects of MTX,[22,23] although other pathways likely contribute to its pleiotropic effects. In general, the safety profile of MTX is viewed as being more favorable than that of other immunosuppressive agents, with several studies showing minimal, if any, increased risk of serious or opportunistic infections.[24] One prospective observational study evaluated the risk of infection in 77 patients with RA treated with MTX compared with 152 patients with RA not on MTX, most of whom were on either no therapy (37%) or sulfasalazine (20%). Sixty-two percent of the MTX group experienced an infection over 1 year, with a relative risk of infection compared with the non-MTX group of 1.52 (95% CI, 1.04–2.22). None of the infectious complications warranted discontinuation of MTX.[25] Differences in the treatment groups may have accounted for the observed increased risk of infection in MTX users, who had significantly worse functional status. Another study of 7971 patients with RA from the Consortium of Rheumatology Researchers of North American (CORRONA) registry, in which MTX and other immunosuppressant treatments were analyzed as time-dependent variables, found an increased rate of infections (eg, urinary tract infection) associated with MTX use (IRR [incidence rate ratio], 1.30; 95% CI, 1.12–1.50) compared with other disease-modifying anti-RA treatments (other than tumor necrosis factor antagonists) but no increase in the risk of opportunistic infections.[26]

A recurring theme with immunosuppression is that combination therapy, although potentially more effective in controlling disease activity, may compound infectious risk. Furthermore, use of multiple therapies concurrently or sequentially complicates clinicians' ability to pinpoint which agent may be the underlying culprit. Many case reports of CNS infections associated with MTX are in the setting of concomitant glucocorticoid or other immunosuppressant use.[27–29]

Data addressing the risk of CNS infection associated with MTX are sparse. However, several neurotoxic side effects of MTX related to the dose and route of administration can mimic CNS infections. High-dose systemic MTX is used for CNS inflammatory syndromes, including some rheumatologic diseases, but confers greater risk of toxicities.[30] Attenuating the neurotoxic effects of MTX is an important management principle that relies on leucovorin rescue when high-dose MTX is used. Some toxicities, such as aseptic meningitis and posterior reversible encephalopathy syndrome, are generally self-limited and do not necessitate treatment beyond holding MTX.[31,32] Others, like MTX-associated myelopathy, warrant prompt cessation of MTX and consideration of folate metabolites.[33]

Cyclophosphamide

Cyclophosphamide (CYC), an alkylating agent with potent antiproliferative activity, was initially developed as a chemotherapeutic drug. Pulse-dose intravenous CYC is used for severe rheumatologic conditions, including lupus nephritis, CNS lupus, and some vasculitides. Bone marrow suppression from high-dose CYC leads to greater susceptibility to infection.[16] However, even in the absence of leukopenia, CYC disrupts both T-cell[34,35] and B-cell function,[36] resulting in impaired cell-mediated and humoral immunity[37] and increased infection risk. As with glucocorticoids, cumulative dose and duration are directly tied to toxicity. As a result, curtailing exposure to CYC with pulse regimens is generally associated with fewer adverse effects, including leukopenia,[38] although it is unclear whether this translates into fewer infectious complications.[39]

CYC is associated with bacterial, viral, and opportunistic infections related to various pathogens.[16] In one retrospective study of 65 rheumatologic patients receiving CYC, infection occurred in 37%, none of which involved the CNS.[40] Risk of infection may be exacerbated by combination therapy because CYC is typically given in conjunction with glucocorticoids. In a controlled trial of 82 patients with lupus nephritis randomized to pulse methylprednisolone, CYC, or combination therapy, approximately 7% of the methylprednisolone group, 25% of the CYC group, and 33% of the combination therapy group had at least 1 infectious complication.[41] Among 100 patients with SLE on CYC and glucocorticoids, infections occurred in 45% of patients receiving combination therapy versus 12% of a separate group of patients with SLE on glucocorticoid monotherapy.[16] Several infections with CNS involvement were documented in patients on CYC, including *Cryptococcus neoformans* and *Nocardia asteroides*. Risk factors for infection were leukopenia nadir less than or equal to 3000/μL and use of sequential intravenous and oral CYC.

Biologic Immunomodulatory Therapies

In contrast with the broadly immunosuppressive agents discussed earlier, biologic therapies for rheumatic diseases are more targeted in hopes of establishing therapeutic efficacy while minimizing off-target complications. Although biologics generally do not cause global immunosuppression, they still modulate immune function and can confer an increased risk of infectious complications. This article focuses on infections of the CNS associated with select, commonly used biologic immunomodulatory agents in the rheumatologists' toolbox.

Tumor necrosis factor inhibitors

Tumor necrosis factor (TNF) is synthesized by various immune cells and is integral to phagosome activation, macrophage differentiation, and granuloma formation and maintenance.[42] Granulomatous infections, including mycobacterial, fungal (eg, cryptococcosis,[43,44] histoplasmosis,[45] coccidiomycosis,[46] aspergillosis,[43] and candidiasis), and parasitic infections (eg, toxoplasmosis[43]) warrant special consideration given the role of TNF in granulomatous reactions.

Tuberculosis (TB) is a well-known infectious complication of TNF antagonists.[47–50] Data are lacking from population-based studies on the incidence of CNS TB associated with TNF inhibitors. Not all TNF inhibitors are equivalent in terms of the risk of reactivation of TB, with etanercept, a soluble TNF receptor fusion protein, carrying a lower risk than the monoclonal TNF antibodies (eg, infliximab, adalimumab).[48] As with TB related to other causes of immunosuppression,[51] patients on TNF inhibitors are more likely to develop extrapulmonary and disseminated disease.[48,52] The most common CNS syndrome of TB is meningitis, which has a tropism for the base of the brain and may be complicated by infarcts and hydrocephalus. Tuberculomas have been described with and without pulmonary involvement in the setting of TNF antagonism.[53–55]

When CNS TB occurs, prompt diagnosis and treatment are critical. Every effort should be made to show definitive microbiological or histologic evidence of tuberculosis.[56] The diagnostic yield of acid-fast bacilli (AFB) examination in CSF ranges from 37% with 1 sampling to as high as 87% with up to 4 serial examinations,[57] although the yield is exceedingly technician dependent and better sensitivities are typically found in high-prevalence settings with exceptionally well-trained and experienced personnel. If initial testing is unrevealing but the suspicion remains high, additional lumbar punctures for cultures and AFB staining should be considered. Clinicians should collect a large volume of CSF (ie, 10 mL) in the final tube to maximize capture of bacilli at the base of the brain and should communicate with the laboratory about the suspected diagnosis to optimize sample processing. CSF mycobacterial nucleic acid amplification testing and adenosine deaminase may add to the diagnostic evaluation.[58] Although the World Health Organization recommends Xpert MTB/Rif (Xpert) testing as the initial diagnostic test for TB from CSF when sample volume is low, and limitations of Xpert for the diagnosis of CNS TB should be recognized.[59] Studies of the use of Xpert MTB/Rif Ultra (Ultra), a next-generation assay that is more sensitive than Xpert, for improved diagnostic accuracy for CNS TB are eagerly awaited.

Screening for and treatment of latent TB infection is an important early risk reduction strategy when using TNF inhibitors. Screening should include exposure history, physical examination, tuberculin skin test, and/or an interferon gamma release assay (IGRA). Patients who are immunosuppressed (including most patients with rheumatologic illness being considered for anti-TNF therapy) without TB risk factors should be screened with an IGRA. For patients with risk factors, 2 screening tests should be performed.[60] An indeterminate IGRA result can be repeated. If screening is positive, further investigation should include chest radiography and sputum examination as indicated, followed by initiation of appropriate treatment. Although screening measures for TB have dramatically decreased the incidence of TB reactivation in the setting of TNF antagonism,[61] the sensitivity of screening tests is imperfect, and TB should always be considered in patients on TNF inhibitors.

Cryptococcus species are encapsulated fungi commonly found in soil and bird droppings. Diagnosis of CNS cryptococcal infection relies on antigen detection and CSF examination and culture. Effective control of increased intracranial pressure (ICP) is critical in the management of cryptococcal meningoencephalitis.[62,63] Even in the absence of clinical evidence of increased ICP,[64] a lumbar puncture should be performed, unless contraindicated, to evaluate the opening pressure, followed by mechanical drainage to reduce the pressure to less than 20 cm H_2O or by roughly 50% if extremely increased.[65] Daily therapeutic lumbar punctures may be required to maintain pressure in the normal range, and surgical drainage with placement of a percutaneous lumbar drain may be appropriate. Acetazolamide and glucocorticoids have not been shown to be effective in the management of increased ICP for human immunodeficiency virus (HIV)–associated cryptococcal meningoencephalitis, and may be harmful.[66,67]

Use of TNF inhibitors also predisposes to infection with endemic mycoses, which can involve the CNS in the form of meningitis, encephalitis, and/or myelitis. Histoplasmosis, which is endemic to the Ohio and Mississippi River Valleys, is the most common fungal infection associated with use of TNF inhibitors[68] and may be more common than TB.[69] As with TB, histoplasmosis infections among patients on TNF inhibitors are generally thought to be more severe and widely disseminated than in immunocompetent patients. In a retrospective study of 98 patients who developed histoplasmosis on TNF inhibitors, with RA as the most common underlying diagnosis, 2 patients (2%) had CNS involvement.[70] Combination therapy with glucocorticoids was a risk factor for greater disease severity. Clinicians should inquire about potential exposures and travel to or residence in endemic areas, as well as symptoms of active or recent infection before initiation of TNF inhibition therapy. Serologic or antigen screening for histoplasmosis in preparation for starting a TNF inhibitor is not recommended.[45] Depending on the severity of the infection, resumption of TNF inhibitor therapy may be considered after treatment and confirmation of undetectable antigen levels.[70] However, careful clinical and laboratory monitoring is recommended.

Coccidioidomycosis and blastomycosis are two other endemic mycoses with CNS manifestations for which patients on TNF inhibitors are at potentially increased risk, although the frequency of these infections is lower than that of histoplasmosis.[68,69] Because CNS coccidioidomycosis requires lifelong therapy, experts recommend against resumption of TNF inhibitor therapy in these patients.[71]

When patients develop mycobacterial or invasive fungal infections, TNF antagonists should be held, and the appropriate antimicrobial regimen initiated. Paradoxic immune reconstitution inflammatory syndrome (IRIS), including of the CNS,[72] can occur when immunosuppression is reduced or discontinued. Ironically, TNF antagonists have been used to treat IRIS, including CNS IRIS, in HIV-infected persons and patients posttransplant, which speaks to the complexities of IRIS and immune modulation associated with TNF inhibition.[73,74] In addition, some complications of TNF antagonism may mimic CNS infection. For example, autoimmune/granulomatous reactions and demyelinating disease have been reported with these agents.[75]

In addition to more common bacterial infections, including bacterial meningitis,[76] the risk of several intracellular pathogens, such as *Listeria* and *Nocardia*, both of which are neurotropic, challenging to diagnose, and associated with high mortality,[77–79] is increased with TNF inhibitors.[80,81] Severe herpesvirus CNS infections have also been reported.[82,83] In one series of TNF inhibitor–associated herpes simplex virus (HSV) encephalitis cases, brain MRI and CSF HSV polymerase chain reaction (PCR) were initially negative in 2 of 3 patients.[84] Although a negative CSF HSV PCR can occur early in HSV encephalitis,[85] empiric antiviral therapy should be continued despite negative testing if clinical suspicion for HSV encephalitis is high, including in patients on TNF inhibitors.

B cell–targeted agents

Rituximab is a chimeric anti-CD20 monoclonal immunoglobulin G1 antibody that depletes peripheral B cells via complement-mediated and antibody-dependent cytotoxicity. Mature plasma cells do not express CD20 and are unaffected by rituximab, as are existing antibody levels.[86] Rituximab is used in the treatment of SLE, RA, and other rheumatic conditions, as well as hematologic malignancies, neuromyelitis optica, and other immune-mediated neurologic conditions.

The precise risk of infection associated with rituximab for patients with rheumatologic disease remains uncertain. Many reported cases of serious infections associated with rituximab are in patients who have received multiple prior biologic and nonbiologic immunomodulatory agents, including TNF antagonists (see case 2). Available data suggest that infectious risk associated with rituximab is lower than with TNF inhibitors and may not be increased in this population, unlike in patients with hematologic malignancies or posttransplant.[87] Unlike with TNF inhibitors, an association between rituximab and increased TB risk has not been shown, and there are no official recommendations to screen for latent TB infection before initiation of rituximab.[88]

The best-recognized opportunistic CNS infection associated with rituximab is progressive multifocal leukoencephalopathy (PML), a demyelinating disease of the CNS caused by infection of oligodendrocytes by reactivated JC virus.[89] The risk of PML in patients with RA treated with rituximab is an estimated 1 per 25,000 patients,[90] considerably lower than in patients with multiple sclerosis on natalizumab,[91] although the mortality may be as high as 90% overall.[92] Although JC virus antibody screening is an integral risk reduction strategy for patients treated with natalizumab, there is currently no role for screening in patients on rituximab.[91,93] Monitoring patients for clinical signs and symptoms of neurologic impairment, including aphasia, visual deficits, and focal weakness, may be a more useful screening tool for emerging PML, which generally has a subacute presentation.

Rituximab can also cause hypogammaglobulinemia, particularly with repeated cycles, predisposing to infections that may require immunoglobulin replacement.[94]

SUMMARY

Rheumatologists should be familiar with the risk of CNS infections associated with broadly immunosuppressive and biologic immunomodulatory agents used to treat rheumatic diseases. Awareness of these infectious complications can help guide screening and prophylaxis, when indicated.

REFERENCES

1. Thomas E, Symmons DP, Brewster DH, et al. National study of cause-specific mortality in rheumatoid arthritis, juvenile chronic arthritis, and other rheumatic conditions: a 20 year followup study. J Rheumatol 2003;30(5):958–65.
2. Zhang G, Zhang L, Duff GW. A negative regulatory region containing a glucocorticosteroid response element (nGRE) in the human interleukin-1beta gene. DNA Cell Biol 1997;16(2):145–52.
3. Scheinman RI, Cogswell PC, Lofquist AK, et al. Role of transcriptional activation of I kappa B alpha in mediation of immunosuppression by glucocorticoids. Science 1995;270(5234):283–6.
4. Tobler A, Meier R, Seitz M, et al. Glucocorticoids downregulate gene expression of GM-CSF, NAP-1/IL-8, and IL-6, but not of M-CSF in human fibroblasts. Blood 1992;79(1):45–51.
5. Rhen T, Cidlowski JA. Antiinflammatory action of glucocorticoids–new mechanisms for old drugs. N Engl J Med 2005;353(16):1711–23.
6. Boumpas DT, Chrousos GP, Wilder RL, et al. Glucocorticoid therapy for immune-mediated diseases: basic and clinical correlates. Ann Intern Med 1993;119(12):1198–208.
7. Paliogianni F, Ahuja SS, Balow JP, et al. Novel mechanism for inhibition of human T cells by glucocorticoids. Glucocorticoids inhibit signal transduction through IL-2 receptor. J Immunol 1993;151(8):4081–9.
8. Lanza L, Scudeletti M, Puppo F, et al. Prednisone increases apoptosis in in vitro activated human peripheral blood T lymphocytes. Clin Exp Immunol 1996;103(3):482–90.
9. Olnes MJ, Kotliarov Y, Biancotto A, et al. Effects of systemically administered hydrocortisone on the human immunome. Sci Rep 2016;6:23002.
10. Klein NC, Go CH, Cunha BA. Infections associated with steroid use. Infect Dis Clin North Am 2001;15(2):423–32, viii.
11. Sakuma Y, Katoh T, Owada K, et al. Initial functional status predicts infections during steroid therapy for renal diseases. Clin Nephrol 2005;63(2):68–73.
12. Strangfeld A, Eveslage M, Schneider M, et al. Treatment benefit or survival of the fittest: what drives the time-dependent decrease in serious infection rates under TNF inhibition and what does this imply for the individual patient? Ann Rheum Dis 2011;70(11):1914–20.
13. Chen JY, Wang LK, Feng PH, et al. Risk of shingles in adults with primary Sjogren's syndrome and treatments: a nationwide population-based cohort study. PLoS One 2015;10(8):e0134930.
14. Dixon WG, Abrahamowicz M, Beauchamp ME, et al. Immediate and delayed impact of oral glucocorticoid therapy on risk of serious infection in older patients with rheumatoid arthritis: a nested case-control analysis. Ann Rheum Dis 2012;71(7):1128–33.

15. Ginzler E, Diamond H, Kaplan D, et al. Computer analysis of factors influencing frequency of infection in systemic lupus erythematosus. Arthritis Rheum 1978; 21(1):37–44.
16. Pryor BD, Bologna SG, Kahl LE. Risk factors for serious infection during treatment with cyclophosphamide and high-dose corticosteroids for systemic lupus erythematosus. Arthritis Rheum 1996;39(9):1475–82.
17. Vargas PJ, King G, Navarra SV. Central nervous system infections in Filipino patients with systemic lupus erythematosus. Int J Rheum Dis 2009;12(3):234–8.
18. Harter JG, Reddy WJ, Thorn GW. Studies on an intermittent corticosteroid dosage regimen. N Engl J Med 1963;269:591–6.
19. Fauci AS. Alternate-day corticosteroid therapy. Am J Med 1978;64(5):729–31.
20. Fauci AS, Dale DC, Balow JE. Glucocorticosteroid therapy: mechanisms of action and clinical considerations. Ann Intern Med 1976;84(3):304–15.
21. Harpaz R, Ortega-Sanchez IR, Seward JF, Advisory Committee on Immunization Practices (ACIP) Centers for Disease Control and Prevention (CDC). Prevention of herpes zoster: recommendations of the Advisory Committee on Immunization Practices (ACIP). MMWR Recomm Rep 2008;57(RR-5):1–30 [quiz: CE32–34].
22. Tian H, Cronstein BN. Understanding the mechanisms of action of methotrexate: implications for the treatment of rheumatoid arthritis. Bull NYU Hosp Jt Dis 2007; 65(3):168–73.
23. Brown PM, Pratt AG, Isaacs JD. Mechanism of action of methotrexate in rheumatoid arthritis, and the search for biomarkers. Nat Rev Rheumatol 2016;12(12): 731–42.
24. McLean-Tooke A, Aldridge C, Waugh S, et al. Methotrexate, rheumatoid arthritis and infection risk: what is the evidence? Rheumatology (Oxford) 2009;48(8): 867–71.
25. van der Veen MJ, van der Heide A, Kruize AA, et al. Infection rate and use of antibiotics in patients with rheumatoid arthritis treated with methotrexate. Ann Rheum Dis 1994;53(4):224–8.
26. Greenberg JD, Reed G, Kremer JM, et al. Association of methotrexate and tumour necrosis factor antagonists with risk of infectious outcomes including opportunistic infections in the CORRONA registry. Ann Rheum Dis 2010;69(2): 380–6.
27. Pulivarthi S, Reshi RA, McGary CT, et al. Cerebral toxoplasmosis in a patient on methotrexate and infliximab for rheumatoid arthritis. Intern Med 2015;54(11): 1433–6.
28. Darley MD, Saad D, Haydoura S, et al. Spinal epidural abscess following minimally invasive dental examination in a rheumatoid arthritis patient receiving methotrexate, glucocorticoids, and anti-tumor necrosis factor therapy. J Clin Rheumatol 2015;21(1):52–3.
29. Trillos RF, Fernandez-Avila DG, Diaz MC, et al. Cryptococcal meningoencephalitis in a patient with rheumatoid arthritis treated with methotrexate and prednisone. Reumatol Clin 2014;10(5):346–7.
30. Beh SC, Kildebeck E, Narayan R, et al. High-dose methotrexate with leucovorin rescue: for monumentally severe CNS inflammatory syndromes. J Neurol Sci 2017;372:187–95.
31. Matsuda M, Kishida D, Kinoshita T, et al. Leukoencephalopathy induced by low-dose methotrexate in a patient with rheumatoid arthritis. Intern Med 2011;50(19): 2219–22.
32. Gonzalez-Suarez I, Aguilar-Amat MJ, Trigueros M, et al. Leukoencephalopathy due to oral methotrexate. Cerebellum 2014;13(1):178–83.

33. Cachia D, Kamiya-Matsuoka C, Pinnix CC, et al. Myelopathy following intrathecal chemotherapy in adults: a single institution experience. J Neurooncol 2015; 122(2):391–8.

34. Bast RC Jr, Reinherz EL, Maver C, et al. Contrasting effects of cyclophosphamide and prednisolone on the phenotype of human peripheral blood leukocytes. Clin Immunol Immunopathol 1983;28(1):101–14.

35. McCune WJ, Golbus J, Zeldes W, et al. Clinical and immunologic effects of monthly administration of intravenous cyclophosphamide in severe systemic lupus erythematosus. N Engl J Med 1988;318(22):1423–31.

36. Cupps TR, Edgar LC, Fauci AS. Suppression of human B lymphocyte function by cyclophosphamide. J Immunol 1982;128(6):2453–7.

37. Clements PJ, Yu DT, Levy J, et al. Effects of cyclophosphamide on B- and T-lymphocytes in rheumatoid arthritis. Arthritis Rheum 1974;17(4):347–53.

38. de Groot K, Harper L, Jayne DR, et al. Pulse versus daily oral cyclophosphamide for induction of remission in antineutrophil cytoplasmic antibody-associated vasculitis: a randomized trial. Ann Intern Med 2009;150(10):670–80.

39. Harper L, Morgan MD, Walsh M, et al. Pulse versus daily oral cyclophosphamide for induction of remission in ANCA-associated vasculitis: long-term follow-up. Ann Rheum Dis 2012;71(6):955–60.

40. Woytala PJ, Morgiel E, Luczak A, et al. The safety of intravenous cyclophosphamide in the treatment of rheumatic diseases. Adv Clin Exp Med 2016;25(3): 479–84.

41. Gourley MF, Austin HA 3rd, Scott D, et al. Methylprednisolone and cyclophosphamide, alone or in combination, in patients with lupus nephritis. A randomized, controlled trial. Ann Intern Med 1996;125(7):549–57.

42. Gardam MA, Keystone EC, Menzies R, et al. Anti-tumour necrosis factor agents and tuberculosis risk: mechanisms of action and clinical management. Lancet Infect Dis 2003;3(3):148–55.

43. Wallis RS, Broder MS, Wong JY, et al. Granulomatous infectious diseases associated with tumor necrosis factor antagonists. Clin Infect Dis 2004;38(9):1261–5.

44. Munoz P, Giannella M, Valerio M, et al. Cryptococcal meningitis in a patient treated with infliximab. Diagn Microbiol Infect Dis 2007;57(4):443–6.

45. Hage CA, Bowyer S, Tarvin SE, et al. Recognition, diagnosis, and treatment of histoplasmosis complicating tumor necrosis factor blocker therapy. Clin Infect Dis 2010;50(1):85–92.

46. Bergstrom L, Yocum DE, Ampel NM, et al. Increased risk of coccidioidomycosis in patients treated with tumor necrosis factor alpha antagonists. Arthritis Rheum 2004;50(6):1959–66.

47. Centers for Disease Control and Prevention (CDC). Tuberculosis associated with blocking agents against tumor necrosis factor-alpha–California, 2002-2003. MMWR Morb Mortal Wkly Rep 2004;53(30):683–6.

48. Tubach F, Salmon D, Ravaud P, et al. Risk of tuberculosis is higher with anti-tumor necrosis factor monoclonal antibody therapy than with soluble tumor necrosis factor receptor therapy: the three-year prospective French Research Axed on Tolerance of Biotherapies registry. Arthritis Rheum 2009;60(7):1884–94.

49. Gomez-Reino JJ, Carmona L, Valverde VR, et al. Treatment of rheumatoid arthritis with tumor necrosis factor inhibitors may predispose to significant increase in tuberculosis risk: a multicenter active-surveillance report. Arthritis Rheum 2003; 48(8):2122–7.

50. Brassard P, Kezouh A, Suissa S. Antirheumatic drugs and the risk of tuberculosis. Clin Infect Dis 2006;43(6):717–22.

51. Aaron L, Saadoun D, Calatroni I, et al. Tuberculosis in HIV-infected patients: a comprehensive review. Clin Microbiol Infect 2004;10(5):388–98.
52. Dixon WG, Hyrich KL, Watson KD, et al. Drug-specific risk of tuberculosis in patients with rheumatoid arthritis treated with anti-TNF therapy: results from the British Society for Rheumatology Biologics Register (BSRBR). Ann Rheum Dis 2010;69(3):522–8.
53. Lynch K, Farrell M. Cerebral tuberculoma in a patient receiving anti-TNF alpha (adalimumab) treatment. Clin Rheumatol 2010;29(10):1201–4.
54. Galati V, Grilli E, Busi Rizzi E, et al. Cerebral tubercular lesions in a patient treated with infliximab for Crohn's disease. J Neurol 2008;255(12):1981–2.
55. Selvarajah L, Choon SE, Tarekh NA, et al. Cerebral tuberculoma with pulmonary tuberculosis in a patient with psoriasis treated with adalimumab, an anti-tumor necrosis factor-alpha agent. Int J Dermatol 2016;55(2):e115–7.
56. Zunt JR, Baldwin KJ. Chronic and subacute meningitis. Continuum (Minneap Minn) 2012;18(6 Infectious Disease):1290–318.
57. Kennedy DH, Fallon RJ. Tuberculous meningitis. JAMA 1979;241(3):264–8.
58. Leonard JM. Central nervous system tuberculosis. Microbiol Spectr 2017;5(2): TNMI7-0044-2017.
59. Bahr NC, Marais S, Caws M, et al. GeneXpert MTB/Rif to diagnose tuberculous meningitis: perhaps the first test but not the last. Clin Infect Dis 2016;62(9):1133–5.
60. Winthrop KL, Weinblatt ME, Daley CL. You can't always get what you want, but if you try sometimes (with two tests–TST and IGRA–for tuberculosis) you get what you need. Ann Rheum Dis 2012;71(11):1757–60.
61. Carmona L, Gomez-Reino JJ, Rodriguez-Valverde V, et al. Effectiveness of recommendations to prevent reactivation of latent tuberculosis infection in patients treated with tumor necrosis factor antagonists. Arthritis Rheum 2005;52(6): 1766–72.
62. Pappas PG. Cryptococcal infections in non-HIV-infected patients. Trans Am Clin Climatol Assoc 2013;124:61–79.
63. Rolfes MA, Hullsiek KH, Rhein J, et al. The effect of therapeutic lumbar punctures on acute mortality from cryptococcal meningitis. Clin Infect Dis 2014;59(11): 1607–14.
64. Graybill JR, Sobel J, Saag M, et al. Diagnosis and management of increased intracranial pressure in patients with AIDS and cryptococcal meningitis. The NIAID Mycoses Study Group and AIDS Cooperative Treatment Groups. Clin Infect Dis 2000;30(1):47–54.
65. Perfect JR, Dismukes WE, Dromer F, et al. Clinical practice guidelines for the management of cryptococcal disease: 2010 update by the Infectious Diseases Society of America. Clin Infect Dis 2010;50(3):291–322.
66. Newton PN, Thai le H, Tip NQ, et al. A randomized, double-blind, placebo-controlled trial of acetazolamide for the treatment of elevated intracranial pressure in cryptococcal meningitis. Clin Infect Dis 2002;35(6):769–72.
67. Beardsley J, Wolbers M, Kibengo FM, et al. Adjunctive dexamethasone in HIV-associated cryptococcal meningitis. N Engl J Med 2016;374(6):542–54.
68. Wallis RS, Broder M, Wong J, et al. Reactivation of latent granulomatous infections by infliximab. Clin Infect Dis 2005;41(Suppl 3):S194–8.
69. Winthrop KL, Yamashita S, Beekmann SE, et al, Infectious Diseases Society of America Emerging Infections Network. Mycobacterial and other serious infections in patients receiving anti-tumor necrosis factor and other newly approved biologic therapies: case finding through the Emerging Infections Network. Clin Infect Dis 2008;46(11):1738–40.

70. Vergidis P, Avery RK, Wheat LJ, et al. Histoplasmosis complicating tumor necrosis factor-alpha blocker therapy: a retrospective analysis of 98 cases. Clin Infect Dis 2015;61(3):409–17.

71. Smith JA, Kauffman CA. Endemic fungal infections in patients receiving tumour necrosis factor-alpha inhibitor therapy. Drugs 2009;69(11):1403–15.

72. Tanaka T, Sekine A, Tsunoda Y, et al. Central nervous system manifestations of tuberculosis-associated immune reconstitution inflammatory syndrome during adalimumab therapy: a case report and review of the literature. Intern Med 2015;54(7):847–51.

73. Scemla A, Gerber S, Duquesne A, et al. Dramatic improvement of severe cryptococcosis-induced immune reconstitution syndrome with adalimumab in a renal transplant recipient. Am J Transplant 2015;15(2):560–4.

74. Sitapati AM, Kao CL, Cachay ER, et al. Treatment of HIV-related inflammatory cerebral cryptococcoma with adalimumab. Clin Infect Dis 2010;50(2):e7–10.

75. Bradshaw MJ, Mobley BC, Zwerner JP, et al. Autopsy-proven demyelination associated with infliximab treatment. Neurol Neuroimmunol Neuroinflamm 2016; 3(2):e205.

76. Kang SJ, Kim HY, Kim YS, et al. Intractable pneumococcal meningoencephalitis associated with a TNF-alpha antagonist. J Neurol Sci 2014;344(1–2):215–8.

77. Bodro M, Paterson DL. Listeriosis in patients receiving biologic therapies. Eur J Clin Microbiol Infect Dis 2013;32(9):1225–30.

78. Bradshaw MJ, Pawate S, Bloch KC, et al. Clinical reasoning: a 52-year-old man with diplopia and ataxia. Neurology 2016;87(13):e140–3.

79. Chow FC, Marson A, Liu C. Successful medical management of a *Nocardia farcinica* multiloculated pontine abscess. BMJ Case Rep 2013;2013 [pii: bcr2013201308].

80. Bowie VL, Snella KA, Gopalachar AS, et al. Listeria meningitis associated with infliximab. Ann Pharmacother 2004;38(1):58–61.

81. Al-Tawfiq JA, Al-Khatti AA. Disseminated systemic *Nocardia farcinica* infection complicating alefacept and infliximab therapy in a patient with severe psoriasis. Int J Infect Dis 2010;14(2):e153–7.

82. Ma C, Walters B, Fedorak RN. Varicella zoster meningitis complicating combined anti-tumor necrosis factor and corticosteroid therapy in Crohn's disease. World J Gastroenterol 2013;19(21):3347–51.

83. Baek W, Lee SG, Kim YS, et al. Fatal varicella-zoster virus vasculopathy associated with adalimumab therapy. Arch Neurol 2012;69(9):1193–6.

84. Bradford RD, Pettit AC, Wright PW, et al. Herpes simplex encephalitis during treatment with tumor necrosis factor-alpha inhibitors. Clin Infect Dis 2009;49(6): 924–7.

85. Bradshaw MJ, Venkatesan A. Herpes simplex virus-1 encephalitis in adults: pathophysiology, diagnosis, and management. Neurotherapeutics 2016;13(3): 493–508.

86. Cambridge G, Leandro MJ, Teodorescu M, et al. B cell depletion therapy in systemic lupus erythematosus: effect on autoantibody and antimicrobial antibody profiles. Arthritis Rheum 2006;54(11):3612–22.

87. Kelesidis T, Daikos G, Boumpas D, et al. Does rituximab increase the incidence of infectious complications? A narrative review. Int J Infect Dis 2011;15(1):e2–16.

88. Buch MH, Smolen JS, Betteridge N, et al. Updated consensus statement on the use of rituximab in patients with rheumatoid arthritis. Ann Rheum Dis 2011;70(6): 909–20.

89. Molloy ES, Calabrese LH. Progressive multifocal leukoencephalopathy associated with immunosuppressive therapy in rheumatic diseases: evolving role of biologic therapies. Arthritis Rheum 2012;64(9):3043–51.
90. Clifford DB, Ances B, Costello C, et al. Rituximab-associated progressive multifocal leukoencephalopathy in rheumatoid arthritis. Arch Neurol 2011;68(9): 1156–64.
91. Borie D, Kremer JM. Considerations on the appropriateness of the John Cunningham virus antibody assay use in patients with rheumatoid arthritis. Semin Arthritis Rheum 2015;45(2):163–6.
92. Carson KR, Evens AM, Richey EA, et al. Progressive multifocal leukoencephalopathy after rituximab therapy in HIV-negative patients: a report of 57 cases from the research on adverse drug events and reports project. Blood 2009;113(20): 4834–40.
93. Clavel G, Moulignier A, Semerano L. Progressive multifocal leukoencephalopathy and rheumatoid arthritis treatments. Joint Bone Spine 2017 [Epub ahead of print].
94. Makatsori M, Kiani-Alikhan S, Manson AL, et al. Hypogammaglobulinaemia after rituximab treatment-incidence and outcomes. QJM 2014;107(10):821–8.

Neurologic Features of Immunoglobulin G4–Related Disease

Mahmoud AbdelRazek, MD[a], John H. Stone, MD, MPH[b],*

KEYWORDS

- Immunoglobulin G4 • Meningeal inflammation • Multiorgan disease
- Orbital myositis • Orbital pseudo tumor • Hypophysitis

KEY POINTS

- IgG4-related disease (IgG4-RD) is an immune-mediated condition that can involve any organ in the body, including the central and peripheral nervous systems.
- The most common neurological features of IgG4-RD result from disease in the orbits, pachymeninges, cavernous sinus, and pituitary gland and stalk.
- Serum IgG4, often found in high concentrations in patients with IgG4-RD, is not believed to play a direct pathophysiological role in mediating tissue injury in most patients with this condition. Rather, the elevated serum IgG4 is believed to be a counter-regulatory mechanism.
- IgG4-RD typically responds well to either glucocorticoid therapy or B cell depletion. However, most patients flare during or after these treatments.

INTRODUCTION

Immunoglobulin (Ig) G4–related disease (IgG4-RD) has been recognized as a discrete, multiorgan condition only since 2003.[1] This immune-mediated disease can affect both the central and peripheral nervous systems, as well as nearly any other organ in the body. The most common neurologic features of IgG4-RD result from disease in the (1) orbits; (2) pachymeninges, including complications of pachymeningeal inflammation within the orbital apex and cavernous sinus; and (3) substance of the pituitary gland and stalk, leading to diabetes insipidus or hypopituitarism; as well as (4) a perineuropathy that can involve either peripheral or cranial nerves. Disease affecting the brain parenchyma is rare but reported. The diagnosis of IgG4-RD is often challenging, requiring careful correlation of pathologic or radiologic findings with the patient's

Disclosure: Dr J.H. Stone has received research grants and performed consulting for Roche (Genentech) in the area of immunoglobulin G4–related disease.
[a] Department of Neurology, Mayo clinic, 200 First Street. SouthWest Rochester, MN 55905, USA; [b] Rheumatology Unit, Massachusetts General Hospital, 55 Fruit Street, Boston, MA 02114, USA
* Corresponding author.
E-mail address: jhstone@mgh.harvard.edu

clinical features. IgG4-RD often mimics malignancy, infection, and other immune-mediated conditions.

IgG4-RD must also be distinguished from a growing number of neurologic diseases in which IgG4 autoantibodies are recognized to play a role in the pathophysiology. Querol and colleagues,[2] 2013, found that in a subset of subjects with chronic inflammatory demyelinating polyneuropathy, for example, pathogenic IgG4 autoantibodies directed against contactin-1, the contactin-1–associated protein-1(CASPR1), or the neurofascin-155 molecules seem to drive the disease.[3] Similarly, beyond the central and peripheral nervous systems, the autoantibodies associated with subsets of pemphigus and idiopathic membranous nephropathy are also primarily of the IgG4 subclass. These diseases are not part of the IgG4-RD spectrum. IgG4-RD is not known to be associated with any specific pathogenic autoantibody identified to date. Rather, it is associated with the infiltration of IgG4+ plasma cells into tissues and, in many patients, dramatic elevations of polyclonal serum IgG4 concentrations. In some cases, nonspecific immune complexes involving IgG4 antibodies may contribute secondarily to tissue injury, but this is not believed to be the primary mechanism of immunologic injury.

GENERAL CLINICAL FEATURES AND COMMON PRESENTATIONS

The presentation of IgG4-RD is typically subacute. Many patients have symptoms and signs for months or even years before the diagnosis is established. True fevers are unusual, but constitutional symptoms such as fatigue and weight loss are common. Many patients have arthralgias and other musculoskeletal symptoms, particularly enthesopathy, but frank arthritis is atypical and suggests other diseases.

IgG4-RD often presents as a mass lesion, regardless of the organ or body area affected: submandibular gland, pancreas, kidney, orbit, pituitary gland, or meninges.[4] Many patients have symptoms of allergy or atopy, for example, allergic rhinitis, nasal polyps, chronic sinusitis, nasal obstruction, and rhinorrhea. Mild to moderate peripheral eosinophilia and serum IgE concentration elevations that sometimes exceed 10 times the upper limit of normal are common. The basis for these atopic features is not understood fully, but processes inherent to IgG4-RD itself rather than to atopy per se seem to contribute to the eosinophilia and IgE elevation.[5,6]

PATHOLOGIC FINDINGS

Both histopathology findings and immunostaining studies are important in establishing the diagnosis, but neither histopathologic nor immunostaining findings are diagnostic of IgG4-RD in and of themselves. Close pathologic mimickers of IgG4-RD include granulomatosis with polyangiitis, inflammatory myofibroblastic tumors, and others. Rigorous assessment of the clinical features, serologic findings, and radiologic manifestations in light of the pathologic evidence is crucial in patient evaluations.

The typical histopathological findings include a dense lymphoplasmacytic infiltrate enmeshed by an irregularly whorled, storiform fibrosis. Obliterative phlebitis and a mild to moderate tissue eosinophilia are also present in a high percentage of cases. The preponderance of plasma cells within a pathologic specimen, usually but not always greater than 40%, is IgG4-positive. Neither the number of IgG4+ plasma cells per high-power field nor the IgG4+ to IgG+ plasma cell ratio is specific for the diagnosis of IgG4-RD. Multiple other conditions can be associated with infiltration of large numbers of IgG4+ plasma cells, emphasizing the importance of integrating these data with information from other parts of the evaluation before coming to conclusions with regard to diagnosis.

PATHOPHYSIOLOGY

Multiple components of the immune system participate in the pathophysiology of IgG4-RD. As previously noted, the IgG4 molecule itself is not believed to play a primary role in IgG4-RD, albeit there may be some contribution of IgG4-containing immune complexes to tissue injury in some cases. On the other hand, interactions between B and T lymphocytes on several levels seem to be involved in the pathophysiology of IgG4-RD. The prevailing disease concept is that both a specific CD4+ cytotoxic T lymphocyte (CTL) and cells of the B lymphocyte lineage (B cells and plasmablasts) are central to the disease. Using this construct, the CD4+ T cells orchestrating the disease are sustained by continuous antigen-presentation by B cells and plasmablasts.[7] Plasmablasts (CD19 + CD38 + CD27 + CD20-cells) are generally elevated in the peripheral blood of patients with IgG4-RD, even in the setting of a normal serum IgG4 concentration.[8] Both CD4+ CTLs and plasmablasts are expanded in an oligoclonal fashion in the peripheral blood.

B cells (contained within germinal centers) and IgG4+ plasma cells are typically located within germinal centers and at the periphery of germinal centers, respectively. In contrast, CD4+ T cells are typically dispersed throughout localized IgG4-RD lesions. These cytotoxic T cells actively secrete granzyme B and perforin, cytotoxic products more commonly associated with CD8+ T cells. The CD4+ CTLs T cells also elaborate interleukin-1, interferon-gamma, and transforming growth factor-beta, all of which may contribute to the fibrosis so characteristic of this disease.

Another CD4+ T lymphocyte, the T follicular helper cell, interacts with B cells both within lymph nodes and in secondary and tertiary lymphoid organs within sites of disease to drive the class switch to IgG4.[9] The ultimate purpose of this class switch may be as a counterbalancing measure to the primary immune response, but this is not known for certain.

SEROLOGY

Among patients with IgG4-RD, the range of serum IgG4 levels is extremely broad. Elevations as high as 40-fold to 50-fold above normal are observed, in contrast, approximately 30% of patients with histopathologically confirmed disease have normal serum IgG4 concentrations.[10] Substantial elevations in serum IgG4 levels are not diagnostic of IgG4-RD in and of themselves but may be extremely important in suggesting the possibility of this diagnosis. The correlation between serum IgG4 concentrations and the need for additional treatment is only approximate, but high serum IgG4 concentrations at baseline identify patients who are unlikely to respond with a sustained remission to a glucocorticoid course of moderate duration.[11]

IgG4 is distinctly different from other IgG subclasses in its ability to undergo dissociation at its hinge region, recombining with other half-antibodies to form bispecific molecules.[12] IgG4 is known to bind the fragment crystallizable (Fc) portion of other immunoglobulins poorly and to be an ineffective activator of the complement cascade under most circumstances. The role of IgG in IgG4-RD may be to serve as an antigen sink at sites of disease, binding loose antigen within inflammatory foci but not inciting further tissue injury.

CLINICAL AND RADIOLOGICAL PRESENTATIONS OF NEUROLOGIC IMMUNOGLOBULIN G4–RELATED DISEASE

Neurologic manifestations of IgG4-RD can be the presenting symptom of the disease.[13–18] IgG4-RD can involve the substance of the dura matter (ie, pachymeninges), pituitary gland and stalk, peripheral nerves, and (rarely) the brain parenchyma. Important neurologic complications also ensue from involvement of structures within the orbit and cavernous sinus.

Two major patterns of neurologic involvement by IgG4-RD are recognized. First, neurologic structures can be affected by direct infiltration of chronic IgG4-related inflammation into the substance of the different anatomic components of the central or peripheral nervous system. Second, neurologic tissues can be compressed by the mass effect of a nearby tissue affected by IgG4-RD.

MENINGEAL DISEASE

IgG4-RD is among the most common causes of nonmalignant meningeal inflammation.[19] IgG4-RD should be considered in cases with unexplained radiographic evidence of pachymeningeal disease, particularly if hypertrophic or nodular. Meningeal IgG4-RD manifests mainly in the pachymeninges (ie, dura mater) of the brain or spinal cord.[20] In a single-center cohort of 125 IgG4-RD subjects, IgG4-related pachymeningitis occurred in 3 (2.4%) subjects.[21]

Symptoms of IgG4-related pachymeningitis depend on the location of the disease, and occur secondary to 1 or more of several mechanisms. First, traction of the dura may lead to headache, typically retro-orbital or frontal when the dura of the anterior and middle cranial fossa is involved. Alternatively, when the dura of the posterior cranial fossa is affected, headaches in the occipital or vertex regions may ensue. Second, meningeal inflammation may encase or compress a nearby structure, typically a cranial nerve, resulting in a cranial neuropathy. Third, blockage of cerebrospinal fluid (CSF) flow may occur, typically at the foramina of Luschka and Magendie, leading to hydrocephalus (**Fig. 1**). A sudden escalation in headache severity should raise a suspicion for the occurrence of hydrocephalus, particularly if there is a positional component to the headaches.

Headache, the most common symptom, can be chronic, intractable, and associated with referred pain to a variety of cranial and facial structures because of dural traction. IgG4-related pachymeningitis involving the dura around the cavernous sinus (**Fig. 2**) can present similarly to Tolosa-Hunt syndrome with proptosis, diplopia, and retrobulbar pain. Other middle cranial fossa dural lesions can present with visual acuity problems or visual field loss due to optic nerve and chiasmal compression.[22] Pachymeningeal disease at the orbital apices can present with diplopia (**Fig. 3**).

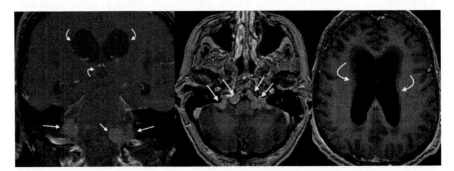

Fig. 1. A 71-year-old white woman with biopsy-proven IgG4-related pachymeningitis. This postcontrast T1 MRI shows ballooning of the lateral and third ventricles (*curved arrows*) likely secondary to obstruction of the foramina of Luschka and Magendi with pachymeningeal disease, seen here thickened and enhancing on MRI (*straight arrows*).

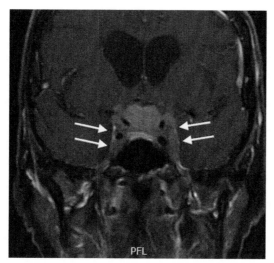

Fig. 2. Postcontrast T1 MRI demonstrating pachymeningeal disease (*arrows*) afflicting both cavernous sinuses.

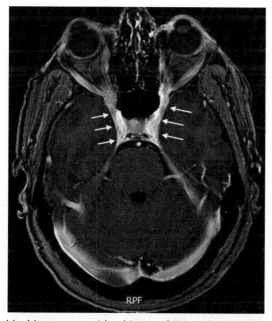

Fig. 3. A 60-year-old white woman with a history of SLE and IgG4-related pachymeningitis diagnosed with meningeal biopsy. This T1-postcontrast MRI shows symmetric pachymeningeal thickening and enhancement (*arrows*) intracranially at the orbital apices, left greater than right. There was slight abduction deficit in the left eye without diplopia but no reduction of visual acuity.

Spinal IgG4-related pachymeningitis may occur in isolation, unaccompanied by other neurologic or non-neurological IgG4-RDs.[14,15,23,24] It can manifest with a syndrome of myelopathy, radiculopathy, or myeloradiculopathy. Depending on location, this can present as neck, midback, or lower back pain that radiates to the limbs; progressive paraparesis or rarely quadriparesis; and/or bladder and bowel dysfunction.

IgG4-related pachymeningitis usually appears radiologically as homogenous dural lesions, diffuse thickening at a single site, or multiple discrete nodules. Computed tomography scans demonstrate IgG4-related pachymeningitis to be isodense compared with brain matter on noncontrast studies. MRI studies reveal these lesions to be hypointense or isointense on noncontrast T1-weighted and T2-weighted imaging.[25,26] Both imaging modalities show homogenous enhancement on postcontrast studies, with lesions that enhance gradually on dynamic studies.[25,26] Both adjacent bone destruction and intralesional calcifications are unusual in patients with IgG4-related pachymeningitis.[25]

CEREBROSPINAL FLUID FINDINGS IN IMMUNOGLOBULIN G4–RELATED PACHYMENINGITIS

The CSF examination can be useful in the assessment of patients with potential IgG4-related pachymeningitis. Patients with IgG4-related pachymeningitis generally have a mild CSF pleocytosis with a lymphocytic predominance. In a series of 10 subjects, the mean (range) of nucleated cells within the CSF was $25/mm^3$ $(22–260 mm^3)$. The CSF protein is also frequently mildly elevated, with a mean (range) of 86 mg/dL (22–260) in the same series.[27] Oligoclonal bands can also occur in the CSF,[28] suggesting intrathecal production of IgG4. Larger numbers of subjects with IgG4-related pachymeningitis need to be studied in a systematic manner, however, before definitive conclusions can be drawn on this point.

One study compared the CSF findings of 3 subjects with IgG4-related pachymeningitis to those of 21 subjects with other causes of hypertrophic pachymeningitis, as well as to those of 9 controls. All 3 of the subjects with IgG4-related pachymeningitis had CSF IgG4 levels greater than 2.27 mg/dL. In contrast, only 5% of those with pachymeningitis of other causes and none of the controls had CSF concentrations this high. A cutoff of 0.47 for IgG4-Loc (an index for intrathecal IgG4 production) correctly categorized all 3 IgG4-related pachymeningitis subjects while misclassifying none of those in the other 2 groups.[28]

ORBITAL DISEASE

Orbital structures that can be affected by IgG4-RD, leading to neurologic manifestations, include (1) the extraocular muscles and levator palpebrae; (2) the optic nerve (cranial nerve II) and ophthalmic artery; (3) the superior and inferior branches of the oculomotor nerve (III), trochlear (IV), frontal (V1), lacrimal (V1) and nasociliary (V1) nerves; and (4) the infraorbital (V2) and zygomatic (V2) nerves.

Inflammation associated with the disease can also infiltrate the extraocular muscles. Extraocular muscle enlargement is usually associated with dacryoadenitis.[29] The orbital soft tissue can also be involved (**Fig. 4**), in isolation or in association with other ocular structures, and typically presents with painless proptosis. Proptosis often occurs secondary to enlargement of any of the ocular adnexa with IgG4-related chronic inflammation, including the lacrimal glands, the extraocular muscles, or the orbital soft tissue itself. In addition, IgG4-RD can cause an orbital pseudotumor that impinges on or encircles the optic nerve. Orbital apex lesions afflicting the optic nerve and causing

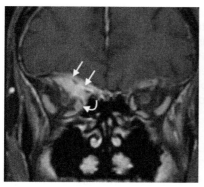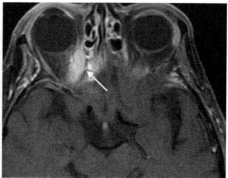

Fig. 4. Right eye orbital soft tissue IgG4-RD (*straight arrows*) displacing the right medial rectus (*curved arrow*) inferiorly.

reduced vision have been described, demonstrated radiologically as enlarged optic nerve sheaths.[30,31]

Radiologic features of IgG4-related orbital disease include predominant involvement of the lateral rectus in terms of frequency and size of enlargement.[32] In a review of 172 cases of IgG4-related ophthalmic disease, the structures most frequently involved on imaging were the lacrimal glands (62%–88%), orbital fat (29%–40%), extraocular muscles (19%–25%), and branches of the trigeminal nerve (10%–39%). Retro-orbital extension to involve the cavernous sinus was observed in 3 of 27 subjects in 1 series.[32]

Inflammatory lesions of IgG4-related orbital disease are more frequently isointense or hypointense on T2 MRI sequencing compared with non–IgG4-RD causes of orbital infiltrative disorders.[33] This hypointensity likely reflects the hypercellularity and fibrosis that is characteristic of IgG4-RD pathologic findings.

PITUITARY GLAND AND STALK DISEASE

IgG4-RD commonly involves the pituitary gland and stalk in what is known collectively as IgG4-related hypophysitis.[20] This can be further classified according to the anatomic structure involved and its ensuing clinical picture into anterior gland disease, posterior gland involvement with stalk disease, and panhypophysitis. Panhypophysitis is the most common presentation of IgG4-RD in this area.[34] IgG4-related hypophysitis occurs commonly as a single-organ manifestation of the disease rather than in the context of multiorgan IgG4-RD.

Hormonal disturbances secondary to hypopituitarism are common in IgG4-related hypophysitis, perhaps more common than in lymphocytic hypophysitis.[35,36] Hypopituitarism has been reported to occur in up to 83%[34,35] of IgG4-related hypophysitis cases, diabetes insipidus in up to 72%,[34,35] and both syndromes in 59% of patients.[34] Patients whose IgG4-RD primarily affects the anterior pituitary gland tend to present with reduced libido, hypogonadism, hypothyroidism, and hypoadrenalism. In contrast, patients with IgG4-RD involvement of the posterior pituitary gland or infundibular stalk present with central diabetes insipidus–related symptoms of polyuria and polydipsia.[37] Patients with panhypophysitis present with a combination of both syndromes. Constitutional symptoms such as headache, fever, weight loss, loss of appetite, lethargy, hypersomnia, and fatigue also occur.

Clinical outcomes are varied. Many patients do not regain pituitary function and require long-term hormonal replacement therapy despite radiographic resolution of the pituitary lesions following treatment. Others, however, return to a functionally normal endocrine status after successful treatment.

MRI demonstrates an enlarged pituitary gland and/or thickened stalk with hypointense T2 lesions that homogenously enhances with gadolinium **(Fig. 5)**.[25,26] Cystic formations inside the enlarged gland can be seen.[34] Subsequently, an empty sella can develop after steroid therapy.[34] Loss of the normal posterior pituitary gland and stalk T1 precontrast hyperintensity is also well described.[25,26,34]

PERIPHERAL NERVE DISEASE

Peripheral nerves can be involved with IgG4-RD by 1 of 2 mechanisms. First, the nerves can become compressed by the mass effect of local IgG4-RD involvement of non-neural tissue.[38] Second, the epineurium may be involved with chronic inflammatory aggregates caused by IgG4-RD, with or without further infiltration into the perineurium.[30,39] Both mechanisms can result in varying degrees of axonal damage with ensuing loss of both large and small myelinated fibers,[39] with or without demyelination. There are no reports of inflammatory IgG4-RD cell infiltration into the endoneurium or nerve fibers on histopathology and thus this loss of axons is likely related to functional trophic changes as a result of chronic inflammation.

Branches of the trigeminal nerve, most characteristically the infraorbital nerve **(Fig. 6)**, are perhaps the most frequently involved peripheral or cranial nerves. Pathologic sections of these involved nerves have demonstrated infiltration of IgG4-RD into the epineurium of the nerve.[30] The finding of infraorbital nerve involvement, however, is usually an incidental finding detected on the performance of head imaging for the evaluation of other IgG4-RD symptomatology. Similarly, asymptomatic spinal nerve root involvement was described in 3 subjects, none of whom had IgG4-RD involving any of the surrounding tissues.[30]

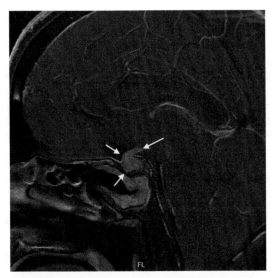

Fig. 5. T1 postcontrast MRI sequence demonstrating homogenous enhancement (*arrows*) of the anterior pituitary gland, posterior gland, and stalk.

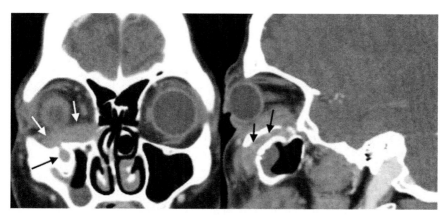

Fig. 6. IgG4-RD involving the right eye orbital soft tissue (*white arrows*) and the right in-fraorbital nerve (*black arrows*) that is thickened and expands the infraorbital canal, seen here on coronal (*right*) and sagittal (*left*) cuts.

CENTRAL NERVOUS SYSTEM PARENCHYMAL DISEASE

The substance of the brain and the spinal cord are rarely involved by IgG4-RD. The authors are aware of only 1 case with satisfactory evidence of brain parenchyma involvement.[40] Otherwise, there are 2 reports of IgG4-related pachymeningitis in which the inflammation extends to involve the underlying brain parenchyma.[16,41] In those 2 cases, although the substance of the brain itself was not biopsied, the proximity of the parenchymal lesions and their concomitant resolution with their associated pachymeningitis after glucocorticoid therapy supports the notion of IgG4-RD pathologic complications. There is also a single account of an intraventricular IgG4-RD mass lesion with sufficient evidence in a 2009 case report,[18] with no further cases of intraventricular IgG4-RD since that time.

TREATMENT

Data on the treatment of IgG4-related neurologic disease are sparse, consisting of only anecdotal reported experiences and small case series. Glucocorticoids are typically the first line of treatment of IgG4-RD, but these agents frequently fail to induce sustained disease remissions in the absence of (or even despite) ongoing treatment.[42] For serious neurologic disease that threatens permanent neurologic injury or death, the authors recommend using rituximab in association with glucocorticoids, based on considerable experience with rituximab for the treatment of non-neurological manifestations of IgG4-RD.[43] It is worth noting, however, for the rare cases of IgG4-RD involving the brain parenchyma, that rituximab does not achieve good central nervous system concentrations in the presence of an intact blood-brain barrier.

REFERENCES

1. Kamisawa T, Funata N, Hayashi Y, et al. A new clinicopathological entity of IgG4-related autoimmune disease. J Gastroenterol 2003;38(10):982–4.

2. Querol L, Nogales-Gadea G, Rojas-Garcia R, et al. Antibodies to contactin-1 in chronic inflammatory demyelinating polyneuropathy. Ann Neurol 2013;73(3): 370–80.

3. Querol L, Nogales-Gadea G, Rojas-Garcia R, et al. Neurofascin IgG4 antibodies in CIDP associate with disabling tremor and poor response to IVIg. Neurology 2014;82(10):879–86.

4. Kamisawa T, Zen Y, Pillai S, et al. IgG4-related disease. Lancet 2015;385(9976): 1460–71.

5. Della Torre E, Mattoo H, Mahajan VS, et al. Prevalence of atopy, eosinophilia, and IgE elevation in IgG4-related disease. Allergy 2014;69(2):269–72.

6. Mattoo H, Della-Torre E, Mahajan VS, et al. Circulating Th2 memory cells in IgG4-related disease are restricted to a defined subset of subjects with atopy. Allergy 2014;69(3):399–402.

7. Mattoo H, Mahajan VS, Maehara T, et al. Clonal expansion of CD4(+) cytotoxic T lymphocytes in patients with IgG4-related disease. J Allergy Clin Immunol 2016; 138(3):825–38.

8. Wallace ZS, Mattoo H, Carruthers M, et al. Plasmablasts as a biomarker for IgG4-related disease, independent of serum IgG4 concentrations. Ann Rheum Dis 2015;74(1):190–5.

9. Maehara T, Mattoo H, Ohta M, et al. Lesional CD4+ IFN-gamma+ cytotoxic T lymphocytes in IgG4-related dacryoadenitis and sialoadenitis. Ann Rheum Dis 2017;76(2):377–85.

10. Carruthers MN, Khosroshahi A, Augustin T, et al. The diagnostic utility of serum IgG4 concentrations in IgG4-related disease. Ann Rheum Dis 2015;74(1):14–8.

11. Wallace ZS, Mattoo H, Mahajan VS, et al. Predictors of disease relapse in IgG4-related disease following rituximab. Rheumatology 2016;55(6):1000–8.

12. Aalberse RC, Stapel SO, Schuurman J, et al. Immunoglobulin G4: an odd antibody. Clin Exp Allergy 2009;39(4):469–77.

13. Rice CM, Spencer T, Bunea G, et al. Intracranial spread of IgG4-related disease via skull base foramina. Pract Neurol 2016;16(3):240–2.

14. Radotra BD, Aggarwal A, Kapoor A, et al. An orphan disease: IgG4-related spinal pachymeningitis: report of 2 cases. J Neurosurg Spine 2016;25(6):790–4.

15. Gu R, Hao PY, Liu JB, et al. Cervicothoracic spinal cord compression caused by IgG4-related sclerosing pachymeningitis: a case report and literature review. Eur Spine J 2016;25(Suppl 1):147–51.

16. Li LF, Tse PY, Tsang FC, et al. IgG4-related hypertrophic pachymeningitis at the falx cerebrii with brain parenchymal invasion: a case report. World Neurosurg 2015;84(2):591.e7-10.

17. Takuma K, Kamisawa T, Igarashi Y. Autoimmune pancreatitis and IgG4-related sclerosing cholangitis. Curr Opin Rheumatol 2011;23(1):80–7.

18. Lui PC, Fan YS, Wong SS, et al. Inflammatory pseudotumors of the central nervous system. Hum Pathol 2009;40(11):1611–7.

19. Wallace ZS, Carruthers MN, Khosroshahi A, et al. IgG4-related disease and hypertrophic pachymeningitis. Medicine 2013;92(4):206–16.

20. Stone JH, Khosroshahi A, Deshpande V, et al. Recommendations for the nomenclature of IgG4-related disease and its individual organ system manifestations. Arthritis Rheum 2012;64(10):3061–7.

21. Wallace ZS, Deshpande V, Mattoo H, et al. IgG4-related disease: clinical and laboratory features in one hundred twenty-five patients. Arthritis Rheumatol 2015; 67(9):2466–75.

22. Behbehani RS, Al-Nomas HS, Al-Herz AA, et al. Bilateral intracranial optic nerve and chiasmal involvement in IgG4-related disease. J Neuroophthalmol 2015; 35(2):229–31.

23. Ezzeldin M, Shawagfeh A, Schnadig V, et al. Hypertrophic spinal pachymeningitis: idiopathic vs. IgG4-related. J Neurol Sci 2014;347(1–2):398–400.
24. Zwicker J, Michaud J, Torres C. IgG4-related disease presenting as dural thickening - a rare cause of myelopathy. Can J Neurol Sci 2014;41(3):392–6.
25. Katsura M, Mori H, Kunimatsu A, et al. Radiological features of IgG4-related disease in the head, neck, and brain. Neuroradiology 2012;54(8):873–82.
26. Toyoda K, Oba H, Kutomi K, et al. MR imaging of IgG4-related disease in the head and neck and brain. AJNR Am J Neuroradiol 2012;33(11):2136–9.
27. Lu LX, Della-Torre E, Stone JH, et al. IgG4-related hypertrophic pachymeningitis: clinical features, diagnostic criteria, and treatment. JAMA Neurol 2014;71(6): 785–93.
28. Della-Torre E, Galli L, Franciotta D, et al. Diagnostic value of IgG4 Indices in IgG4-related hypertrophic pachymeningitis. J Neuroimmunol 2014;266(1–2): 82–6.
29. Wallace ZS, Deshpande V, Stone JH. Ophthalmic manifestations of IgG4-related disease: single-center experience and literature review. Semin Arthritis Rheum 2014;43(6):806–17.
30. Inoue D, Zen Y, Sato Y, et al. IgG4-related perineural disease. Int J Rheumatol 2012;2012:401890.
31. Plaza JA, Garrity JA, Dogan A, et al. Orbital inflammation with IgG4-positive plasma cells: manifestation of IgG4 systemic disease. Arch Ophthalmol 2011; 129(4):421–8.
32. Tiegs-Heiden CA, Eckel LJ, Hunt CH, et al. Immunoglobulin G4-related disease of the orbit: imaging features in 27 patients. AJNR Am J Neuroradiol 2014; 35(7):1393–7.
33. Soussan JB, Deschamps R, Sadik JC, et al. Infraorbital nerve involvement on magnetic resonance imaging in European patients with IgG4-related ophthalmic disease: a specific sign. Eur Radiol 2016;27(4):1335–43.
34. Bando H, Iguchi G, Fukuoka H, et al. The prevalence of IgG4-related hypophysitis in 170 consecutive patients with hypopituitarism and/or central diabetes insipidus and review of the literature. Eur J Endocrinol 2014;170(2):161–72.
35. Caputo C, Bazargan A, McKelvie PA, et al. Hypophysitis due to IgG4-related disease responding to treatment with azathioprine: an alternative to corticosteroid therapy. Pituitary 2014;17(3):251–6.
36. Caturegli P, Lupi I, Landek-Salgado M, et al. Pituitary autoimmunity: 30 years later. Autoimmun Rev 2008;7(8):631–7.
37. Hattori Y, Tahara S, Ishii Y, et al. A case of IgG4-related hypophysitis without pituitary insufficiency. J Clin Endocrinol Metab 2013;98(5):1808–11.
38. Takahashi M, Shimizu T, Inajima T, et al. A case of localized IgG4-related thoracic periarteritis and recurrent nerve palsy. Am J Med Sci 2011;341(2):166–9.
39. Ohyama K, Koike H, Iijima M, et al. IgG4-related neuropathy: a case report. JAMA Neurol 2013;70(4):502–5.
40. Regev K, Nussbaum T, Cagnano E, et al. Central nervous system manifestation of IgG4-related disease. JAMA Neurol 2014;71(6):767–70.
41. Kim EH, Kim SH, Cho JM, et al. Immunoglobulin G4-related hypertrophic pachymeningitis involving cerebral parenchyma. J Neurosurg 2011;115(6):1242–7.
42. Khosroshahi A, Wallace ZS, Crowe JL, et al. International consensus guidance statement on the management and treatment of IgG4-related disease. Arthritis Rheumatol 2015;67(7):1688–99.
43. Carruthers MN, Topazian MD, Khosroshahi A, et al. Rituximab for IgG4-related disease: a prospective, open-label trial. Ann Rheum Dis 2015;74(6):1171–7.

Involvement of the Peripheral Nervous System in Polyarteritis Nodosa and Antineutrophil Cytoplasmic Antibodies–Associated Vasculitis

John B. Imboden, MD

KEYWORDS

- Antineutrophil cytoplasmic antibodies (ANCA) • Granulomatosis with polyangiitis
- Microscopic polyangiitis
- Eosinophilic granulomatosis with polyangiitis (Churg-Strauss syndrome)
- Polyarteritis nodosa • Mononeuritis multiplex • Ischemic neuropathy

KEY POINTS

- Peripheral nerve involvement is common in polyarteritis nodosa and the antineutrophil cytoplasmic antibodies (ANCA)-associated vasculitides, particularly eosinophilic granulomatosis with polyangiitis (Churg-Strauss syndrome).
- The underlying mechanism is arteritis of the vasa nervorum, leading to ischemic neuropathy.
- The classic presentation is stepwise involvement of 1 or more named peripheral nerves in the setting of weeks or more of antecedent constitutional symptoms.

OVERVIEW

Polyarteritis nodosa (PAN) and the antineutrophil cytoplasmic antibodies (ANCA)-associated vasculitides commonly affect the peripheral nervous system, especially early in the course of disease. Neuropathies develop in most (65%–85%) patients with PAN.[1] Among the ANCA-associated vasculitides, peripheral nerve involvement is more prevalent in eosinophilic granulomatosis with polyangiitis (EGPA), occurring in upwards of 80% of cases, than in microscopic polyangiitis (MPA) and occurs least often in granulomatosis with polyangiitis (GPA) (~25%).[2–6] The shared mechanism is vasculitis of the vasa nervorum, the small nutrient arteries that supply peripheral nerves, leading to nerve ischemia.[1–8] The classic clinical presentation is acute or

Dr J.B. Imboden has no disclosures and no conflicts of interest.
Department of Medicine, University of California, Box 0868, San Francisco, CA 94143, USA
E-mail address: john.imboden@ucsf.edu

Rheum Dis Clin N Am 43 (2017) 633–639
http://dx.doi.org/10.1016/j.rdc.2017.06.011
0889-857X/17/© 2017 Elsevier Inc. All rights reserved.

subacute mononeuritis multiplex-stepwise involvement of 2 or more named nerves, leading to motor and sensory deficits in the distribution of the affected nerves.[1–8] Pain is common and usually severe.[1,9,10] Additive ischemic insults to multiple nerves can produce diffuse, but often asymmetric, sensory and motor deficits.[1,9,10] Uncommon manifestations include distal sensory neuropathy, radiculopathies, and lumbar or brachial plexopathies.[1–11]

PATHOLOGIC FINDINGS

After entering the nerve, the vasa nervorum branch into complex, anastomosing microvascular networks that run primarily within the epineurium, the connective tissue that surrounds peripheral nerves and also occupies the interfascicular space.[1] PAN and the ANCA-associated vasculitides cause a necrotizing arteritis of vessels within the epineurium and rarely affect the perineurial and endoneurial vessels.[1,2,5,6,9,10] Histologic features of affected vessels include focal fibrinoid necrosis, transmural inflammation, luminal occlusion, and recanalization.[1,2,5,6,9,10] The inflammatory infiltrates usually are mixed, composed of both mononuclear cells and neutrophils.[1,2,5,6,9,10] Eosinophils are prominent in vasculitis due to EGPA.[2,5] Necrotizing arteritis is often segmental, and the involved segments can be a short as 50 microns in length.[1,10] Evidence of ischemic neuropathy is always present, but the severity of the ischemic changes varies.[1,10] Ischemia induces axonal degeneration. Features suggestive of ischemic neuropathy include asymmetry of involvement between and within fascicles and axonal degeneration that is predominantly within the central region of fascicles.[1,10] True nerve infarction is uncommon on biopsy samples of affected sural and superficial peroneal nerves, likely due in part to the segmental nature of the arteritis and to the plexus-like nature of the epineurial circulation, which protects against ischemic injury (ie, the nerves are protected against infarction because epineurial vessels are not necessarily end arteries).[1,10]

CLINICAL SYNDROMES

The peripheral nervous system can be the first organ system affected in PAN and the ANCA-associated vasculitides, particularly EGPA and MPA.[1–6] However, antecedent constitutional symptoms such as weight loss, fatigue, malaise, and low-grade fever usually have been present for weeks to several months.[1–6] The onset of the neuropathy is often abrupt with pain, sensory loss, and weakness in the distribution of 1 (mononeuritis) or more (mononeuritis multiplex) named peripheral nerves (**Table 1**).[1,9,10] The pain is severe and more often described as throbbing or aching than burning. The peroneal nerve is most often affected, followed by the tibial, ulnar, median, and radial nerves.[1,9,10] Involvement can progress in a stepwise to affect additional nerves over weeks to months. Multiple nerves, however, can be affected simultaneously, or the progression of the neuropathy can be rapid, leading to a generalized multifocal neuropathy that may require careful examination to demonstrate that the process is asymmetric.[1,9,10] Uncommon manifestations of systemic arteritis include distal symmetric sensory neuropathies, polyradiculopathies, plexopathies, and purely motor neuropathies.[9–11]

DIAGNOSIS

Systemic vasculitis should always be the primary diagnostic consideration when mononeuritis or mononeuritis multiplex develops in the setting of a systemic illness. The history and physical examination often provide important clues about the correct

Table 1
Peripheral nerve involvement in polyarteritis nodosa and antineutrophil cytoplasmic antibodies vasculitis

Peripheral Nerve	Reported Frequency of Clinical Involvement[1-11]	Characteristic Motor Deficits[25]	Characteristic Sensory Deficits[25]
Peroneal	57%–96%	Dorsiflexion of the foot Dorsiflexion of toes and great toe	Web between 1st and 2nd toes (deep peroneal) Lateral calf and dorsum of foot (common peroneal)
Tibial	11%–86%	Plantar flexion of foot Inversion of foot Flexion of toes and great toe	Sole of the foot
Ulnar	24%–75%	Adduction of the thumb Adduction & abduction of the index finger Abduction of the little finger	Lateral hand, including small finger & lateral aspect of ring finger
Radial	4%–50%	Extension & adduction of the hand at the wrist Extension of the fingers at the metacarpophalangeal joints Supination of the forearm	Dorsal aspect of the thumb and hand proximal to the 2nd and 3rd metacarpophalangeal joints
Median	9%–58%	Pronation of the forearm Flexion and abduction of the hand at the wrist Abduction of the thumb	Palmar surface of the hand from the wrist to the thumb, index and long fingers Dorsal surface of the index and long fingers distal to the metacarpophalangeal joints

specific diagnosis. For example, PAN associated with hepatitis B virus usually develops 6 to 9 months following the episode of acute hepatitis.[12] Mesenteric involvement in PAN is common and can cause postprandial periumbilical pain (abdominal angina); renal arteritis can manifest as new-onset hypertension.[12] A long history of asthma points to the possibility of EGPA, particularly following the recent addition of leukotriene receptor antagonist.[13] Chronic sinus inflammation, nasal ulcerations, scleritis, and serous otitis media suggest GPA.[14] Diffuse alveolar hemorrhage in GPA and MPA may be confused with pneumonia, particularly if hemoptysis is absent or minimal.[14,15]

Virtually all patients with active PAN and ANCA-associated vasculitis have evidence of systemic inflammation as reflected in elevations in the erythrocyte sedimentation rate and the serum level of C-reactive protein and a mild to moderate thrombocytosis.[12–15] Routine laboratory studies can point to clinically silent involvement of other organ systems (eg, glomerulonephritis). Chest radiographs can reveal nodules in GPA, evidence of diffuse alveolar hemorrhage in MPA or GPA, and fleeting infiltrates in EGPA.[13–15]

There are no specific serologic studies for PAN. Positive tests for rheumatoid factors are common but are nonspecific. Serum complement levels can be either low or normal. All patients with hepatitis B–associated PAN have detectable hepatitis B surface antigen. Conventional angiography of affected mesenteric, hepatic, or renal arteries can demonstrate microaneurysms in PAN-findings that are diagnostic in the proper clinical context.[12]

Patients with suspected GPA, MPA, or EGPA should be tested for the presence of ANCA using indirect immunofluorescence on fixed neutrophils and immunoassay for antibodies to proteinase-3 (PR3) and myeloperoxidase (MPO).[16] The sensitivity of ANCA testing for patients with generalized, active GPA or MPA ranges from 78% to 96% but is less in cases of limited GPA or in the early phases of MPA.[16] The sensitivity of ANCA testing for EGPA is only 50%.[2–5] Among patients presenting with vasculitic neuropathy, the sensitivity of ANCA testing is approximately 75% in cases of GPA and MPA, and less than 50% in patients with EGPA.[2–6] The specificity of anti-PR3 antibodies for GPA is significantly higher (greater than 90%) than the specificity of anti-MPO antibodies for MPA or EGPA.[16]

ELECTRODIAGNOSTIC STUDIES

Nerve conduction studies typically demonstrate abnormalities consistent with an axonal neuropathy that affects 1 or more nerves and which often is more extensive than clinically suspected.[1,8–11] The most common findings are low-amplitude compound muscle action potentials and low-amplitude sensory nerve action potentials with normal or only mild slowing of conduction velocity.[1,8–11] Although conduction blocks usually suggest nerve entrapment or acute focal demyelination, occasionally focal ischemic injury causes conduction blocks due to wallerian degeneration and axonal damage or pseudoconduction blocks, which may be misinterpreted as a mixed axonal and demyelinating neuropathy.[1,8–11] Electromyography of distal muscles often demonstrates abnormalities (fibrillations, positive sharp waves) consistent with denervation.[1,8–11]

NERVE BIOPSY

Biopsies of either the sural nerve or the superficial peroneal nerve are standard procedures in the evaluation of a patient with suspected vasculitic neuropathy and can be diagnostic.[1–11] Biopsies may be positive even when nerve conduction studies are normal.[1,8–11] Estimates of the sensitivity of biopsy range from 45% to 70%; therefore, the failure to demonstrate vasculitis on nerve biopsy should never be the sole basis for excluding the diagnosis of vasculitic neuropathy.[1,8–11] Because of the segmental nature of the vasculitis, serial sections of the tissue blocks should be performed. Concomitant biopsy of the gastrocnemius or the peroneus brevis muscles can increase the yield by up to 15%.[1,8–11]

DIFFERENTIAL DIAGNOSIS

The clinical presentations of neuropathy due to PAN and ANCA-associated vasculitides, although often distinctive, are not specific for these disorders. The differential diagnosis includes other diseases that can cause vasculitis of the vasa nervorum: notably nonsystemic vasculitic neuropathy, systemic rheumatic diseases, and mixed cryoglobulinemia.[1,9,10] The vasculopathy associated with long-standing diabetes mellitus, often a mimic of systemic vasculitis, can manifest as mononeuritis multiplex. Compression neuropathies at multiple sites can mimic mononeuritis multiplex; the clinical context and nerve conduction studies point to the correct diagnosis in such cases.[1,9,10] Nerve conduction studies can differentiate ischemic neuropathy from demyelinating disorders, such as Guillain-Barre syndrome, whose clinical presentations sometimes mimic peripheral nerve involvement due to vasculitis.[1,8–11,17]

Nonsystemic vasculitic neuropathy is a vasculitis of the vasa nervorum that has a predilection for the epineural vessels and produces nerve ischemia.[18,19] Clinically, it behaves like an organ-specific vasculitis affecting peripheral nerves; some patients have subclinical perivascular inflammation in skin and muscle.[18,19] The mean age of onset is approximately 60 years, and the female to male ratio is 5 to 4.[18] In contrast to PAN and the ANCA-associated vasculitides, constitutional symptoms are often absent, and the onset is more often chronic and progressive than acute.[18,19] The most common pattern at presentation is an asymmetric polyneuropathy.[18,19] Only a few patients present with mononeuritis multiplex; distal symmetric polyneuropathy is uncommon but well recognized.[18,19]

Vasculitic neuropathies can complicate vasculitis associated with mixed cryoglobulinemia (either essential or due to hepatitis C) but are rare in large vessel vasculitis (giant cell arteritis, Takayasu arteritis) and in Henoch-Schonlein purpura.[1] Longstanding seropositive rheumatoid arthritis (RA) can be associated with a necrotizing arteritis that is indistinguishable from PAN and then can manifest as mononeuritis multiplex.[20] This complication of RA, which occurred in less than 1% of RA patients when it was first described in the 1960s, is now rare. Vasculitic neuropathies are well-recognized complications of systemic lupus erythematosus, primary Sjögren syndrome, scleroderma, and dermatomyositis.[1] Mononeuritis multiplex is an uncommon to rare manifestation of sarcoidosis, leprosy, angiocentric lymphoma, and paraneoplastic syndromes.[1,21–23]

TREATMENT AND OUTCOMES

The underlying disease dictates the treatment regimens for vasculitic neuropathies associated with either PAN or the ANCA-associated vasculitides.[1,9,10,24] Glucocorticoids, initially in high dose, are the mainstay of treatment of PAN, but approximately 50% of patients with PAN also receive cyclophosphamide (administered either in monthly intravenous pulses or as a daily oral dose) for severe or refractory disease.[12] Initial treatment regimens for ANCA-associated vasculitis use high-dose glucocorticoids in combination with rituximab, a B cell-depleting monoclonal antibody, or with cyclophosphamide.[13–15] The response of peripheral neuropathies is variable, but some level of neuropathic pain or motor weakness is common, especially in cases when mononeuritis multiplex has advanced before the initiation of treatment.[1,9,10,24]

REFERENCES

1. Vrancken A, Said G. Vasculitic neuropathy. Handb Clin Neurol 2013;115:463--83.
2. Nagashima T, Cao B, Takeuchi N, et al. Clinicopathological studies of peripheral neuropathy in Churg-Strauss syndrome. Neuropathology 2002;22:299–307.
3. Cottin V, Bel E, Bottero P, et al. Revisiting the systemic vasculitis in eosinophilic granulomatosis with polyangiitis (Churg-Strauss) A study of 157 patients by the Groupe d'Etudes et de Recherche sur les Maladies Rares Pulmonaires and the European Respiratory Taskforce on eosinophilic granulomatosis with polyangiitis (Churg-Strauss). Autoimmun Rev 2017;16:1–9.
4. Cattaneo L, Chierici E, Pavone L, et al. Peripheral neuropathy in Wegener's granulomatosis, Churg-Strauss syndrome, and microscopic polyangiitis. J Neurol Neurosurg Psychiatry 2007;78:1119–23.
5. Guillevin L, Cohen P, Gayraud M, et al. Churg-Strauss syndrome clinical study and long-term follow-up of 96 patients. Medicine (Baltimore) 1999;78:26–37.
6. Guillevin L, Durand-Gasselin B, Cevallos R, et al. Microscopic polyangiitis clinical and laboratory findings in eight-five patients. Arthritis Rheum 1999;42:421–30.
7. Mouthon L, Dunogue B, Guillevin L. Diagnosis and classification of eosinophilic granulomatosis with polyangiitis (formerly named Churg-Strauss syndrome). J Autoimmun 2014;48-49:99–103.
8. Hawke SHB, Davies L, Pamphlett R, et al. Vasculitic neuropathy a clinical and pathological study. Brain 1991;114:2175–90.
9. Gorson KC. Vasculitic neuropathies: an update. Neurologist 2007;13:12–9.
10. Said G, Lacroix C. Primary and secondary vasculitic neuropathy. J Neurol 2005; 252:633–41.
11. Allan SG, Towla HMA, Smith CC, et al. Painful brachial plexopathy: an unusual presentation of polyarteritis nodosa. Postgrad Med J 1982;58:311–5.
12. Stone JH. Polyarteritis nodosa. Current diagnosis and treatment rheumatology. 3rd Edition. New York: McGraw Hill; 2013. p. 285–90.
13. Stone JH. Eosinophilic granulomatosis with polyangiitis (Churg-Strauss syndrome). Current diagnosis and treatment rheumatology. 3rd edition. New York: McGraw Hill; 2013. p. 280–4.
14. Stone JH. Granulomatosis with polyangiitis (Wegener granulomatosis). Current diagnosis and treatment rheumatology. 3rd Edition. New York: McGraw Hill; 2013. p. 264–72.
15. Seo P, Stone JH. Microscopic polyangiitis. Current diagnosis and treatment rheumatology. 3rd Edition. New York: McGraw Hill; 2013. p. 273–9.
16. Csernok E, Moosig F. Current and emerging techniques for ANCA detection in vasculitis. Nat Rev Rheumatol 2014;10:494–501.
17. Huda S, Krshnana A. An unusual case of mononeuritis multiplex. Pract Neurol 2013;13:39–41.
18. Collins MP, Perquet-Collins I. Nonsystemic vasculitis neuropathy: update on diagnosis, classification, pathogenesis, and treatment. Front Neurol Neurosci 2009; 26:26–66. In Pourmand R (ed) Immune-Mediated Neuromuscular Diseases. Basel, Karger.
19. Kararizou E, Davaki P, Karandreas N, et al. Nonsystemic vasculitis neuropathy: a clinicopathological study of 22 cases. J Rheumatol 2005;32:853–8.

20. Schneider HA, Yonker RA, Katz P, et al. Rheumatoid vasculitis: experience with 13 patients and review of the literature. Semin Arthritis Rheum 1985;14:280–6.
21. Mattie R, Irwin RW. Neurosarcoidosis presenting as mononeuritis multiplex. Am J Phys Med Rehabil 2014;03:349–54.
22. Roux S, Grossin M, De Bandt M, et al. Angiotropic large cell lymphoma with mononeuritis multiplex mimicking systemic vasculitis. J Neurol Neurosurg Psychiatry 1995;58:363–6.
23. Martin AC, Friedlander M, Kiernan MC. Paraneoplastic mononeuritis multiplex in non-small-cell lung carcinoma. J Clin Neurosci 2006;13:595–8.
24. Mathew L, Talbot K, Love S, et al. Treatment of vasculitis peripheral neuropathy: a retrospective analysis of outcome. QJM 2007;100:41–51.
25. Medical Research Council. Aids to the examination of the peripheral nervous system. London: Her Majesty's Stationary Office; 1976.

UNITED STATES POSTAL SERVICE ® Statement of Ownership, Management, and Circulation (All Periodicals Publications Except Requester Publications)

1. Publication Title	2. Publication Number	3. Filing Date
RHEUMATIC DISEASE CLINICS OF NORTH AMERICA	006 – 272	9/18/2017

4. Issue Frequency	5. Number of Issues Published Annually	6. Annual Subscription Price
FEB, MAY, AUG, NOV	4	$335.00

7. Complete Mailing Address of Known Office of Publication (Not printer) (Street, city, county, state, and ZIP+4®)

ELSEVIER INC.
230 Park Avenue, Suite 800
New York, NY 10169

Contact Person: STEPHEN R. BUSHING
Telephone (Include area code): 215-239-3688

8. Complete Mailing Address of Headquarters or General Business Office of Publisher (Not printer)

ELSEVIER INC.
230 Park Avenue, Suite 800
New York, NY 10169

9. Full Names and Complete Mailing Addresses of Publisher, Editor, and Managing Editor (Do not leave blank)

Publisher (Name and complete mailing address)

ADRIANNE BRIGIDO, ELSEVIER INC.
1600 JOHN F KENNEDY BLVD. SUITE 1800
PHILADELPHIA, PA 19103-2899

Editor (Name and complete mailing address)

LAUREN BOYLE, ELSEVIER INC.
1600 JOHN F KENNEDY BLVD. SUITE 1800
PHILADELPHIA, PA 19103-2899

Managing Editor (Name and complete mailing address)

PATRICK MANLEY, ELSEVIER INC.
1600 JOHN F KENNEDY BLVD. SUITE 1800
PHILADELPHIA, PA 19103-2899

10. Owner (Do not leave blank. If the publication is owned by a corporation, give the name and address of the corporation immediately followed by the names and addresses of all stockholders owning or holding 1 percent or more of the total amount of stock. If not owned by a corporation, give the names and addresses of the individual owners. If owned by a partnership or other unincorporated firm, give its name and address as well as those of each individual owner. If the publication is published by a nonprofit organization, give its name and address.)

Full Name	Complete Mailing Address
WHOLLY OWNED SUBSIDIARY OF REED/ELSEVIER, US HOLDINGS	1600 JOHN F KENNEDY BLVD. SUITE 1800 PHILADELPHIA, PA 19103-2899

11. Known Bondholders, Mortgagees, and Other Security Holders Owning or Holding 1 Percent or More of Total Amount of Bonds, Mortgages, or Other Securities. If none, check box ► ☐ None

Full Name	Complete Mailing Address
N/A	

12. Tax Status (For completion by nonprofit organizations authorized to mail at nonprofit rates) (Check one)
The purpose, function, and nonprofit status of this organization and the exempt status for federal income tax purposes:
☒ Has Not Changed During Preceding 12 Months
☐ Has Changed During Preceding 12 Months (Publisher must submit explanation of change with this statement)

13. Publication Title	14. Issue Date for Circulation Data Below
RHEUMATIC DISEASE CLINICS OF NORTH AMERICA	MAY 2017

PS Form **3526**, July 2014 [Page 1 of 4 (see instructions page 4)] PSN: 7530-01-000-9931 PRIVACY NOTICE: See our privacy policy on www.usps.com.

---

15. Extent and Nature of Circulation

		Average No. Copies Each Issue During Preceding 12 Months	No. Copies of Single Issue Published Nearest to Filing Date
a. Total Number of Copies (Net press run)		337	260
b. Paid Circulation (By Mail and Outside the Mail)	(1) Mailed Outside-County Paid Subscriptions Stated on PS Form 3541 (Include paid distribution above nominal rate, advertiser's proof copies, and exchange copies)	143	123
	(2) Mailed In-County Paid Subscriptions Stated on PS Form 3541 (Include paid distribution above nominal rate, advertiser's proof copies, and exchange copies)	0	0
	(3) Paid Distribution Outside the Mails Including Sales Through Dealers and Carriers, Street Vendors, Counter Sales, and Other Paid Distribution Outside USPS®	79	67
	(4) Paid Distribution by Other Classes of Mail Through the USPS (e.g. First-Class Mail®)	0	0
c. Total Paid Distribution (Sum of 15b (1), (2), (3), and (4))		222	190
d. Free or Nominal Rate Distribution (By Mail and Outside the Mail)	(1) Free or Nominal Rate Outside-County Copies included on PS Form 3541	42	70
	(2) Free or Nominal Rate In-County Copies Included on PS Form 3541	0	0
	(3) Free or Nominal Rate Copies Mailed at Other Classes Through the USPS (e.g. First-Class Mail)	0	0
	(4) Free or Nominal Rate Distribution Outside the Mail (Carriers or other means)	0	0
e. Total Free or Nominal Rate Distribution (Sum of 15d (1), (2), (3) and (4))		42	70
f. Total Distribution (Sum of 15c and 15e)		264	260
g. Copies not Distributed (See Instructions to Publishers #4 (page 3))		73	0
h. Total (Sum of 15f and g)		337	260
i. Percent Paid (15c divided by 15f times 100)		84.09%	73.08%

* If you are claiming electronic copies, go to line 16 on page 3. If you are not claiming electronic copies, skip to line 17 on page 3.

16. Electronic Copy Circulation

	Average No. Copies Each Issue During Preceding 12 Months	No. Copies of Single Issue Published Nearest to Filing Date
a. Paid Electronic Copies ►	0	0
b. Total Paid Print Copies (Line 15c) + Paid Electronic Copies (Line 16a) ►	222	190
c. Total Print Distribution (Line 15f) + Paid Electronic Copies (Line 16a) ►	264	260
d. Percent Paid (Both Print & Electronic Copies) (16b divided by 16c × 100) ►	84.09%	73.08%

☒ I certify that 50% of all my distributed copies (electronic and print) are paid above a nominal price.

17. Publication of Statement of Ownership

☒ If the publication is a general publication, publication of this statement is required. Will be printed in the NOVEMBER 2017 issue of this publication. ☐ Publication not required.

18. Signature and Title of Editor, Publisher, Business Manager, or Owner

[signature] STEPHEN R. BUSHING - INVENTORY DISTRIBUTION CONTROL MANAGER   Date 9/18/2017

I certify that all information furnished on this form is true and complete. I understand that anyone who furnishes false or misleading information on this form or who omits material or information requested on the form may be subject to criminal sanctions (including fines and imprisonment) and/or civil sanctions (including civil penalties).

PS Form **3526**, July 2014 (Page 3 of 4) PRIVACY NOTICE: See our privacy policy on www.usps.com

Moving?

Make sure your subscription moves with you!

To notify us of your new address, find your **Clinics Account Number** (located on your mailing label above your name), and contact customer service at:

Email: journalscustomerservice-usa@elsevier.com

800-654-2452 (subscribers in the U.S. & Canada)
314-447-8871 (subscribers outside of the U.S. & Canada)

Fax number: 314-447-8029

Elsevier Health Sciences Division
Subscription Customer Service
3251 Riverport Lane
Maryland Heights, MO 63043

*To ensure uninterrupted delivery of your subscription, please notify us at least 4 weeks in advance of move.

Printed and bound by CPI Group (UK) Ltd, Croydon, CR0 4YY

08/05/2025

01864703-0007